FAMILY CAREGIVERS
ON THE JOB

Moving beyond ADLs and IADLs

FAMILY CAREGIVERS ON THE JOB

Moving beyond ADLs and IADLs

Carol Levine
Editor

United Hospital Fund of New York

Library of Congress Cataloging-in-Publication Data

Family caregivers on the job : moving beyond ADLs and IADLs /
Carol Levine, editor.

    p. ;   cm.

Includes bibliographical references and index.

ISBN 1-881277-73-9

1. Caregivers.

[DNLM: 1. Caregivers—standards. 2. Home Nursing—methods.
3. Activities of Daily Living. 4. Outcome and Process Assessment (Health
Care)—methods. WY 200 F1968 2004] I. Levine, Carol. II. United
Hospital Fund of New York.

    RA645.3.F37 2004

    362′.0425—dc22

                        2004006906

ISBN: 1-881277-73-9

For information, write, Publications Program, United Hospital Fund of New York, 350 Fifth Avenue, 23rd Floor, New York, NY 10118-2399.

Contents

Foreword

MORE THAN 27 million family caregivers in the United States provide care to seriously ill or disabled family members at home. Through the efforts of the United Hospital Fund and many other organizations, the issue of family caregiving is making its way onto the national agenda.

But for all the increased attention that the issue has received in recent years, we still have no good way of fully describing or accurately measuring what family caregivers actually do, what it is that makes their work rewarding or challenging, and what help they might need to continue. Absent this knowledge, we cannot begin to design the educational and support services that might spell the difference between satisfaction and burnout, fulfillment and despair. Instead, we continue to rely on Activities of Daily Living (ADLs) and Instrumental Activities of Daily Living (IADLs)—tools developed to measure care *recipients'* functional deficits—to assess the realities of the lives of their family care *providers.*

This volume captures a year's worth of fruitful debate among experts convened from around the country to analyze the limitations of ADLs and IADLs and to explore alternatives. The project was sponsored by the United Hospital Fund, with grant support from The Robert Wood Johnson Foundation.

Since 1996, the United Hospital Fund—a health services research and philanthropic organization whose mission is to shape positive change in health care—has focused on family caregivers. Under the leadership of Carol Levine, an ethicist and herself a family caregiver, the Fund has supported the development of model programs in hospitals, analyzed the burdens on family caregivers, and advocated for supportive public policies. Perhaps most stirringly, it has given voice to family caregivers, at conferences and in books like *The Cultures of Caregiving: Conflict and Common Ground among Families, Health Professionals, and Policy Makers* (Johns Hopkins University Press, 2004) and *Always on Call: When Illness Turns Families into Caregivers* (2nd edition, Vanderbilt University Press, 2004).

We believe that this book can move the discussion about family caregivers to the next level, by identifying the tools needed to develop the kinds of programs that would be most helpful to them. We thank the participants in the yearlong project, the authors, and The Robert Wood Johnson Foundation for its support.

JAMES R. TALLON, JR.
President
United Hospital Fund

Preface

FAMILY CAREGIVING is and always has been the bedrock of society's concern for its ill, disabled, and fragile members. Strong and caring societies encourage strong and caring families, which express their loyalty, obligations, and affection in countless ways. An industrialized, efficiency-oriented, and quantitative society like the United States, however, actually does count the ways in which some people need care and others provide it. Beginning in the 1960s, the universally accepted basic measures for analysis have been the care recipient's needs for assistance in activities of daily living (ADLs), such as bathing, and instrumental activities of daily living (IADLs), such as transportation, and by extension, the family caregiver's job in meeting those needs.

These measures are largely unknown to caregivers themselves. It is hard to imagine a support group, Internet chat group, counseling session, or even a conversation among family members talking about ADLs or IADLs, even though the content may in fact cover some of the items in the measures. Even then, caregivers talk about their tasks in quite different and often highly personal ways that do not appear in research reports or policy proposals. Professionals talk about a person with "three ADLs" or "only IADL needs"; caregivers do whatever needs to be done, whenever it needs to be done.

This book began as a project of the United Hospital Fund's Families and Health Care Project to explore whether ADLs and IADLs suffice as the lingua franca of caregiving policy, research, and professional practice, given the changes in health care financing, medical care, and demographics that have occurred in the past decades. The project convened a working group that approached the challenge of re-examining some basic assumptions in their respective fields with diligence, passion, and creativity. The Robert Wood Johnson Foundation supported the year-long project and provided additional support for the publication of its primary product—this volume. For the foundation's generous support, and especially the thoughtful guidance of Nancy Fishman, Senior Project Officer, we are truly grateful.

The book contains six chapters, each introduced by a summary. Carol Levine and Andrea Hart describe caregiving tasks from caregivers' perspectives, drawing on both the professional literature and caregiver narratives. The ADL-IADL measures, it quickly becomes clear, fail to capture much of the range of difficulty of performing a specific task and do not cover at all some of the most demanding aspects of caregiving, such as navigating the health care system or providing emotional support. Susan Reinhard then traces the development of the ADL-IADL measures from their original purpose in describing the functional deficits of patients to their current all-purpose use in caregiver policy and research. She describes the proliferation of measures and their limitations even for their original purpose. Lynn Friss Feinberg analyzes the important but inconsistent and infrequent use of caregiver assessments that should underlie the provision of education, support, and other forms of assistance. Steven Albert proposes a new framework for describing caregiving, one that takes into account not just what the care recipient needs but also the environment in which caregiving takes place and the cooperation or lack of it from the care recipient. From a policy perspective, Bruce Vladeck cautions that any measure will of necessity be a blunt instrument, and that a long-term change will be difficult to implement. He offers several short-term policy changes that would make a difference. Finally, David Gould reviews the project and its conclusions, with a view toward seeking realizable next steps. An appendix contains an article reprinted from the journal *Generations*, which summarizes the views of the first four chapters.

As the book's editor, one of its authors, and a family caregiver, I want to thank all those who participated as authors or members of the working group. They diligently accepted the challenge of re-examining some basic assumptions of their fields and provided important suggestions. They contributed more than can be acknowledged in this brief preface.

CAROL LEVINE
June 2004

Acknowledgments

IN ADDITION TO the authors in this volume, the participants in the meetings were:

Emily K. Abel, University of California at Los Angeles
Barbara Berkman, School of Social Work, Columbia University
Pamela Doty, U.S. Department of Health and Human Services,
    Office of the Assistant Secretary for Planning and Evaluation
Penny Hollander Feldman, Center for Home Care Policy and
    Research, Visiting Nurse Service of New York
Myra Glajchen, Department of Pain Medicine and Palliative
    Care, Beth Israel Medical Center, New York
Gladys Gonzalez-Ramos, School of Social Work, New York
    University
Ruby H. Greene, RHG Consulting Services
Eileen Hanley, Supportive Care Program, Saint Vincent's Medical
    Center
Gail Gibson Hunt, National Alliance for Caregiving
Rosalie A. Kane, LIC Center, Division of Health Services Research
    and Policy, University of Minnesota School of Public Health
Mary Jane Koren, The Commonwealth Fund
Korbin Liu, Health Policy Center, The Urban Institute
Mary Mittelman, Silberstein Aging and Dementia Research Cen-
    ter, New York University Medical School
Sidney Stahl, Behavioral and Social Research Program, National
    Institute on Aging

Although the authors drew freely from suggestions and comments in revising the papers prepared for the meetings, the participants bear no responsibility for the views expressed in the various chapters.

In addition, several United Hospital Fund staff participated in the sessions:

Phyllis Brooks, Vice President and Director of Communications
David Gould, Senior Vice President for Program
Deborah Halper, Vice President and Director of Education and
    Program Initiatives
Alene Hokenstad, Project Director
Sally Rogers, Senior Vice President for Communications and
    Development
Fredda Vladeck, Project Director, Aging in Place Initiative

Andrea Hart, Program Associate for the Families and Health Care Project, and Shoshana Vasheetz coordinated the meetings. Phyllis Brooks skillfully guided the transformation of the papers into a book.

1

Doing Whatever Needs to Be Done: Caregivers' Perspectives on ADLs and IADLs

Carol Levine and Andrea Hart

SUMMARY

In research and policy arenas, family caregiving is generally described in terms of providing assistance for the care recipient in the activities of daily living (ADLs) and instrumental activities of daily living (IADLs). Although for some caregiving situations the ADL and IADL measures are "good enough," they fail to capture the reality of many, and probably a growing number of, caregivers' responsibilities. Developed for a different purpose, in a different health care and economic environment, these measures are so entrenched as markers of caregiving that they are taken for granted and seldom reconsidered.

Drawing from the professional literature and caregiver narratives, this chapter first reviews the ADL and IADL measures in terms of the kinds of difficulties these deceptively simple tasks often present to caregivers. For example, bathing—a basic ADL—becomes challenging and even dangerous when the care recipient is immobile or demented.

Next the authors describe tasks and activities that are not captured by the ADL and IADL measures or that are so deeply embedded in them that they are unexamined. Some of these tasks and activities are pain management, providing high-tech medical care at home, negotiating the health care system, and managing paid home care aides.

Many caregivers describe what they do in terms of multiple, overlapping roles. When they are overwhelmed with the tasks of caregiving, it becomes difficult to fulfill their primary obligation—providing the emotional support that only they can give. Nor can they take care of themselves or their other obligations to family, job, and community.

RESEARCH ON "informal caregivers"—the family members and friends who provide most of the unpaid long-term care to elderly or disabled individuals—began after the enactment of Medicare and Medicaid in 1965 and accelerated in the mid-1980s and 1990s. The literature on family caregiving is enormous—over 7,000 articles turned up in a recent PubMed search and Barnes&Noble.com lists over 700 books, mostly how-to and inspirational volumes in addition to those for professionals. The research literature is full of important data and insights, especially about caregiver burden and, more recently, rewards. It is surprising, nevertheless, how little ethnographic or "thick" description of caregiving exists.* This gap is partially being filled with a growing number of caregiver narratives.

What does caregiving actually entail? And what are the best ways to describe and understand it? As Susan Reinhard (Chapter 2) shows, since the early 1980s, the tasks of family caregiving have been described in surveys, research studies, and policy decisions as the mirror image of a care recipient's functional deficits. These deficits are categorized as needs for assistance in performing ADLs or IADLs (Katz

---

*This is not the only gap. Ferrell's (2001) review of 50 nursing textbooks' coverage of end-of-life care found that 71 percent had no content at all related to family caregivers. Only 42 of the 45,683 pages concerned family caregivers.

et al. 1963; Lawton and Brody 1969). Although there are several versions of these measures, ADLs typically include aspects of personal care, such as bathing, dressing, eating, toileting, transferring from bed to chair, and walking across the room. IADLs are the activities that involve maintaining a household and interacting with the external world: cooking, cleaning, shopping, housekeeping, driving a car or using public transportation, using the telephone, and managing finances. Managing medication is typically included in this category, though it seems misplaced, since it is so closely related to personal care (Pearson 2000).

In this view, the caregiver's role is to assist the care recipient in accomplishing the basic tasks of daily life he or she used to be able to perform alone and now cannot because of illness or disability, or was never able to do alone because of lifelong disability. The ADL-IADL measures offer a straightforward picture of caregiving, appealing in their simplicity and ease of quantification. They make comparisons possible across groups of caregivers and over time. However, they present a traditional picture of caregiving as the performance of homely domestic chores, or "women's work" (Allen et al. 1993, S209), with the possible exception of managing financial affairs. Good caregiving, according to this scheme, does not seem very different from ordinary living. Shopping, doing housework, preparing meals, helping an elderly person bathe and get dressed—these are or should be part of everyday family life.

In some ways any focus on tasks misses the core of caregiving. As Abel (1990, 141) points out, "The chores that family and friends perform do not exist in a vacuum; rather, they are embedded in intimate personal relationships." Jansson, Nordberg, and Grafstrom (2001, 805) believe that the "activities of daily living or instrumental care . . . divert attention from much work caregivers are engaged in and render them invisible." For this reason, Schumacher and colleagues (2000) assert that caregiving should not be defined solely in terms of tasks and procedures. Nevertheless, we cannot understand the whole of caregiving unless we accurately describe what caregivers do, and how that varies in different situations.

The spectrum of caregiving includes very modest, relatively unchallenging tasks, as well as those that are identical to nursing-home, and in some instances even hospital-based, care. Although for some caregiving situations the ADL-IADL measures are "good enough," they fail to capture the reality of many, and probably a growing number of, caregivers' responsibilities. Developed for a different purpose, in a different health care and economic environment, these measures are so entrenched as markers of caregiving that they are taken for granted and seldom reconsidered.

This chapter begins that reconsideration and points the way toward a deeper and more complex view of caregiving tasks as seen by the people who perform them. It is not a comprehensive literature review but a selection of examples that come from both the professional literature and caregiver narratives. These examples are vivid but not unique. In the first of two main sections, we review the ADL-IADL measures in terms of the kinds of difficulties caregivers face and the skills required to perform them. In the second, we describe tasks and activities that are not captured by the ADL-IADL measures, or are so deeply embedded in them that they are unexamined. These responsibilities are integral to the experience of caregiving.

Inevitably there is some overlap and some indistinct boundaries. Real life is not as clear-cut as sociometric measures might lead us to believe. Caregivers do not think of what they do in terms of performing ADLs and IADLs; they do whatever needs to be done. Then they watch and wait until the next thing needs to be done, and the next, and the next. If, as Woody Allen famously said, "80 percent of success in life is showing up," then 80 percent of success in caregiving may be not only showing up but staying on. Just "being there," of course, means not being able to be anywhere else.

The Reality Behind ADL-IADL Measures

ADLs; or, How Hard Can It Be to Give Mom a Bath?

Sometimes health care professionals—and even some caregivers themselves—compare the personal tasks involved in caring for an ill or disabled person to caring for a baby or young child. "Your mother changed your diapers for you, why can't you do the same for her?" they chide the reluctant new caregiver. However, the situations are quite different. In contrast to traditional "parent-child caregiving that usually results in the independence and self-sufficiency of the child, family caregivers of older persons face the discouraging inevitable deterioration of the care recipient, leading ultimately to death or nursing home placement" (Council on Scientific Affairs 1993, 1283). Added to this reality are the psychological ramifications of role reversal for both caregiver and care recipient (Karlin, Bell, and Noah 2001).

Bathing, toileting, and dressing. In the national and New York City survey of family caregivers conducted by the Harvard School of Public Health, the United Hospital Fund, and the Visiting Nurse Service of New York (VNSNY) (Levine et al. 2000), the two ADLs that were most likely to trigger all the others, and IADLs as well, were bathing and toileting (or in this survey's terminology, "managing incontinence"). A care recipient who needed help in one or both of these tasks was likely to be unable to perform the others.

Bathing is an important health measure to prevent infection, as well as a (formerly) pleasurable one and, by controlling body odor, a social one (Sloane et al. 1995). Yet bathing is clearly one of the most difficult tasks, particularly if the care recipient is demented or has mobility problems (Rader and Barrick 2000). It may be as apparently simple as standing by in case help is needed, or as complicated as moving a paralyzed person from bed to shower chair and into the bathroom, making sure he or she is fully washed and dried, and re-peating the process back to bed.

Even the simplest situation, as the following description shows, can make the caregiver tense with anxiety.

> She [the author] handed him the towel and stood by. She stood wary in the knees to spring forward and catch him should he fall. She an-ticipated which way he might lean, veer, subside. She mustn't spare a blink to look out the window, she might miss the necessary sig-nal of his shifting. . . . Should his right knee buckle now, he'd be less able to stop the fall with the good hand, might crack his chin bone on the sink. She readied catching muscles deep in her feet, calf, torso. This kind of work, readiness, gave less satisfaction than actually do-ing something. How could she complain? She wasn't even a hard-core caregiver, yet. (Strong 1997, 326)

The caregiver may encounter disruptive behavior, particularly when the care recipient feels confused, threatened, or insulted, or if he or she is physically uncomfortable (Rader and Barrick 2000; Sloane et al. 1995). The care recipient may perceive certain acts, such as being moved into the bathroom, undressed, and washed, as physical or sex-ual abuse and may respond with combative behavior (Sloane et al. 1995). If the care recipient suffers from arthritis or other mobility prob-lems, he or she may resist going into the bathroom because move-ment is discomforting and painful.

The caregiver must be very cautious in handling the body of a frail elderly person. As a person ages, the body deteriorates and loses its re-siliency and elasticity, and bones are more prone to fractures and breaks. One caregiver (Pisetsky 1998, 869) reported: "My father had no muscles. Coarse skin covered bones that were held together by ten-dons that seemed frayed and rigid. I was afraid that I would pull off a limb if I lifted him wrong." Dressing a person in this fragile state, or one who is paralyzed, is a challenge requiring not only strength but also an understanding of body mechanics. Special clothing may be necessary. Once a routine is established, the care recipient may not tolerate any deviations from it.

When bathing, the caregiver must monitor verbal and physical gestures for potential signs of pain. To the caregiver and care recipient alike, bathing may seem like a battle rather than a boon. There are many ways to avoid or reduce these anxieties, including bed baths, providing a comforting environment, checking the water and bathroom temperature, organizing all the needed materials ahead of time, using assistive devices and aids, speaking in a soothing voice, and playing music on the radio (Sloane et al. 1995). But, as the Harvard-United Hospital Fund-VNSNY survey (Levine et al. 2000) shows, most caregivers are not given any training in ADLs.

Moreover, most homes are not like hospitals or nursing homes, which have special facilities for showers. Whatever a caregiver has observed or been taught in such a facility is not easy to replicate at home. The level of difficulty in bathing a home-bound person is often equal to that of bathing a nursing home resident. The description in Rader and Barrick (2000) of what certified nurse assistants should do to bathe a resident properly is applicable to the family caregiver as well. The individualized shower care plan the authors present for Mrs. S (see pp. 31–32) is revealing in its myriad details and cautions.

While bathing is a complex process that may take two hours to complete, it usually need not be done every day and may happen only once a week. Toileting, however, is a frequent, almost nonstop task. "Toileting" may indeed be just that—helping a person get to the toilet on time, and making sure that he or she is clean and dry. But even this can be difficult. One caregiver wrote: "Sometimes diarrhea takes him by surprise. When that happens, I clean up floors or sheets or the inside of Jockey shorts while he goes to the roll-in shower to wash off his frustration along with his soiled body" (Anonymous 2000). Although, technically, laundry, as housework, falls in the IADL category, this comment makes it clear that the time and energy devoted to laundry is vastly increased if the care recipient is incontinent. And if the caregiver has to use a laundromat, this task can also be inconvenient and expensive.

"Toileting" for a person in a wheelchair often means limiting options for outings, as another caregiver explained:

> Yes, we do go out to lunch, or a haircut or a dentist appointment, but it is always a gamble whether there will be barriers or a transfer will go smoothly. Excursions either with [my] spouse or on [my] own are usually confined to 2–3 hours (the time between trips to the bathroom). We usually can only use the one at home, because the equipment needed is there. We do not use indwelling catheters so must use toilet facilities. Public restrooms are not usually feasible. We need to be home for meals, bedtimes, toilet times, just to be there—in case. (Drucker 1998)

"Toileting" may not involve the toilet at all, if the care recipient is incontinent of urine or bowels. The care recipient must use indwelling catheters, condom catheters, or adult diapers, which require the caregiver's help in changing and cleaning up. While incontinence can indeed be managed, again, caregivers are typically not given any instruction on how best to do it, the required methods of infection control, and where to find the most appropriate supplies. Skin breakdown is a constant threat for an incontinent person, and monitoring for this problem is a daily chore.

Eating.   While bathing, dressing, and toileting are the most intimate types of ADL, preparing food for and feeding an ill person can also be difficult. He or she may need to eat at a different time from the rest of the family, particularly when taking prescribed medication that must be taken with food.

Many ill people require special diets, for which the caregiver must shop for specific items, prepare meals in precise ways, and often encourage the care recipient to eat what is probably not his or her food of choice. The care recipient may like certain foods at one point and later develop a distaste for them (Schumacher et al. 2000).

Some persons with disabilities may be able to feed themselves, or require only some assistance with cutting pieces of meat; many require feeding by hand, which can be a time-consuming and frustrating process. "Every week [one caregiver] prepares 21 meals for her husband that she stocks in the freezer. It takes an hour to feed him each one" (Fein 1994).

It is not uncommon for a person suffering from a chronic or terminal disease to develop dysphagia, that is, difficulty swallowing (Dunn 1994). Swallowing problems increase the risk that pieces of food will get into the lungs and cause aspiration pneumonia. To prevent this from happening, the caregiver may have to prepare a limited menu that is easy for the care recipient to swallow and to monitor eating so that only small amounts are ingested at a time. As with bathing, an activity that once was a source of pleasure and socialization may become a contest of wills.

The importance of food to well-being and normality are seldom acknowledged (Manthrope and Watson 2003). Eating out is not enjoyable for either care recipient or caregiver when restaurant staff are not helpful or respectful, or when the care recipient's behavior is embarrassing (Manthrope, Watson, and Stimpson 2002). Some caregivers refuse to be intimidated by unpleasant reactions; others simply stay home.

Mobility. Some of the most apparent declines in elderly people's functioning show up in their ability to move and walk (Iezzoni 2003). One caregiver (Ball 1997, 133) recalled: "I remember my shock upon seeing my mother walk with a cane for the first time, a temporary concession to an ambush by the enemy arthritis. . . . Accommodating an aging parent presents just such a series of startling and undignified 'firsts'; . . . the firsts often get worse, not better: canes become walkers,

walkers become wheelchairs, wheelchairs become gurneys in nursing homes."

Moving an immobilized person can also be a daunting and dangerous task. Having to constantly lift dead weight places massive strain on the lifter's back and may lead to the onset of health problems. One caregiver (quoted in Fein 1994) noted, "Moving my husband from the bed, to the commode, to the chair, I just completely threw my back out and needed a chiropractor. . . . That really got me down, because I am very healthy and suddenly it was hard for me to move."

In many facilities immobilized persons are known as "two-person transfers," that is, staff members should not attempt this maneuver alone. Yet at home there are seldom two people always on hand to do the job. One caregiver (Doubrava 1998) related: "[He] requires two young and strong people to lift him from bed to wheelchairs. I am seventy-six-years-old, have emphysema and asthma and have a twenty-pound limit on lifting. . . . When [he] fell or slid to the floor at night, I slept on the floor with him. . . . He was 205 pounds and 5'11" against my 124 pounds and 5'."

Mintz (2002, 94) described a situation in which her husband, who has multiple sclerosis, fell:

> I used a sheet to drag him from the bathroom, across the wooden floor and down the hall, past the guest room and his office, and then onto the carpeting in the master bedroom. There was no place at all in the bathroom that he could hold on to and from which I could try to bend his legs and position them in such a way that, working together, we could maneuver him into a standing position. At least in our bedroom there was a bed frame with decorative cutouts that work well as handholds. . . . The whole process took about forty-five exhausting minutes to go a distance of just twenty-three feet. Steven's skin was rubbed raw and my back was pretty sore.

Even if a care recipient is not moved out of bed but is only turned, the caregiver can strain his or her back. Nursing standards dictate that the position of such a patient be changed every two hours to prevent skin breakdown. While meeting this standard may be possible (but highly unlikely) in a hospital, it is impossible for most family caregivers. Nevertheless, they are often given this instruction when they leave the hospital.

IADLs; or, How Hard Can It Be to Make Telephone Calls?

Compared with the intense, intimate, and often demanding physical nature of ADLs, IADLs may seem easy. In some situations no special training or adaptations are required, and the emotional component of caregiving is minimized. This distinction may explain why, traditionally (and even now, but to a lesser degree), ADLs have been performed by women and IADLs by men.

Even IADL tasks that do not present big challenges individually can collectively take a great deal of the caregiver's time (Bakas, Lewis, and Parsons 2001) and require lifestyle adjustments. One male caregiver (Schindler 1996, 6–7) wrote, "The first week was a crisis period for me, since I felt that I had to juggle a host of obligations and responsibilities. It had come on more suddenly than I had expected. . . . Regular meals had to be provided, visits to the doctor, spending time and occupying him."

Of all the IADLs, shopping seems the least problematic; as long as one has some familiarity with a grocery store, it would seem easy enough to add on a few more trips or a few more items. However, many of the items the care recipient needs—special, often expensive, foods or incontinence supplies, as well as assistive devices, such as special spoons and forks—are not ones that consumers typically buy or know where to find. If the family's overall budget is limited, the family caregiver has to set priorities about the purchase of particular items.

The importance to caregivers of learning how to be good consumers is seldom recognized and the skill of good consumerism is hardly ever taught. Often caregivers must go to the Internet, catalogs, or specialty shops for items that are not carried locally. This effort is time-consuming and frequently frustrating. The situation is even more daunting when the care recipient needs a piece of large, expensive durable medical equipment, such as a wheelchair or hospital bed (Levine and Kuerbis 2001).

Driving a car or using public transportation.   Transportation is an essential IADL. As adults age, vision impairments may hamper their ability to perform certain actions, such as driving. Vision impairments make it difficult to judge distance and to see at night (Cobb and Coughlin 2000). Illness may also cause weakness and lack of coordination.

With the onset of dementia, family caregivers seek to encourage, persuade, or insist that driving is no longer an option. Providing alternate modes of transportation means that the caregiver has to drive the care recipient everywhere he or she needs or wants to go, including to doctors' offices, stores, and other places in the community. A survey of caregivers of patients with lung cancer found that adult children rated transportation as the most time-consuming task, while spouses rated it as the second (providing emotional support was first) (Bakas, Lewis, and Parsons 2001).

As Cobb and Coughlin (2000, 202) point out, "reduced physical flexibility and strength may make getting in and out of a car more difficult." Today's automobiles are not designed for people with mobility problems, and specially outfitted vans are extremely expensive. If it is difficult to get a person out of bed and into a wheelchair, it is close to impossible to get him or her into a regular car.

Many wheelchairs and walkers fold for placement in the trunk of a car, but managing this operation, as the following description suggests, involves careful positioning and planning.

> She [the author] opened the door and walked around to open his and while he maneuvered himself to a standing position, she

opened the back door and pulled out his half walker. She spread his legs, pressed down on the stabilizing bar, snapped it into place, and set it near his good hand. She walked around the car to lock her door with the master key, and joined him for the walk into the restaurant: one foot, walker, other foot, walker, one foot, walker, other foot, walker. . . . Inside, there was the trek across the carpeted floor, its trickiness, its hidden slopes. When he was seated, she ran back to the car, parked it, and returned. (Strong 1997, 331)

In many areas, public transportation systems are not equipped to meet the mobility demands of older adults (Cobb and Coughlin 2000). Some cities have kneeling buses, wheelchair-accessible buses or subways, or paratransit systems (ambulettes or taxis), but such systems may not be available or may be extremely limited for people living in suburban or rural areas.

Even where public paratransit systems and ambulettes are available, they are notoriously unreliable. Depending on the system, a 24-hour or three-to-seven-day advance reservation may be required. The passenger is not guaranteed an on-time arrival or departure, and the trip may also include other passengers whose destinations make the route indirect and longer than it would otherwise be. Private ambulette service is expensive and has many of the same problems.

Using the telephone. When an elderly or cognitively impaired person does not have the functional capacity to operate a telephone (look up numbers, dial, answer the telephone), the family caregiver initiates calls or answers the telephone. If telephone calls were limited to chats with friends and family, or other routine calls, life would be relatively simple. Most caregivers, however, view "making telephone calls" as extended and repeated discussions on behalf of the family member. Many of these calls are with health care professionals to schedule appointments, check on test results, report symptoms, or reorder prescriptions. Many are to public or private payers, to find out whether a service will be reimbursed, to find out why reimbursement was denied when it was initially approved, to check on bills that do not reflect services rendered, or to complain about service on prior calls.

A typical caregiver might respond to the question, What is so hard about making telephone calls? with the following scenario drawn from the author's (CL) own experience:

> Call the paratransit service, wade through the automated messages, wait on hold, finally speak to an operator who informs me that the trip I want to schedule cannot be accommodated. Call the doctor's office to change the appointment to accommodate transportation. On the day of the appointment, call to find out why the ambulette is late. Call the ambulette service from the doctor's office to say that the doctor has been delayed, and so the return trip will also be delayed. Call again to find out when it will be possible to pick up the passenger. And so on, until, often hours later, the trip is completed.

The telephone is a lifeline, but for a caregiver, it can also be a noose.

Managing finances.   For many caregivers and care recipients, taking over money management can be fraught with tension and ambivalence. Many older people are unwilling to tell their adult children (or even their spouses) about their financial status, whether their assets are many or few. Usually, however, once a care recipient's inability to manage money becomes apparent, perhaps through a crisis occasioned by a failure to pay a bill, this IADL will fall to a family member, who must manage everything from sorting out batches of unopened medical bills to paying household expenses.

Managing money requires mathematical, record-keeping, and critical analysis skills and the ability to make judgments about priorities. Where resources are limited and expenses high, managing money can be overwhelming. In addition to the regular household accounting, the illness or disability adds costs for supplies, medications, and a host of other items not covered by public or private insurance.

Medicare provides only limited home health care, and to be eligible for Medicaid a care recipient must be at poverty level and have very few assets. If the care recipient is not eligible for home health care, the family caregiver and other family members take on the financial responsibility to provide home health care, entailing not only financial obligations but also an additional bookkeeping chore. Fein (1994) describes a typical situation: "When she is at work, Ms. ——— pays for a health aide to stay with her mother, using money from her mother's pension and her father's estate. She is usually gone from 8 a.m. to 8:30 p.m., and pays the aide's wages of $7 an hour herself because her mother is ineligible for Medicaid."

Another caregiver (Zeigler 1990, 19) described her experiences with a spouse who had been struck by a drunk driver:

> After two years, my husband's insurance had expired. It is now time to make another move. The nursing home where he was had a long list of residents waiting for Medicaid beds. I applied at numerous facilities and was told . . . they didn't have the Medicaid beds available. What I did was the only thing I knew to do at the time. I quit my job and brought my husband home. I had now become the primary caregiver of my husband. As there was no insurance, my funds were diminishing rapidly. Medicare would not kick in for another eight months. I was praying that he would not have to have any major surgery during that time, so I could survive financially. I had no idea how or when I could go back to work because of his many needs. I had become his physical therapist, speech therapist, occupational therapist, nurse, and wife—not necessarily all in that order.

A spousal caregiver may encounter yet another dilemma if he or she is required alone to manage the family's finances that were previously handled by or with the care recipient. Learning to balance a checkbook or making sure the household bills are paid can be an overwhelming task for anyone who has never had to think about such things. The caregiver has to learn to become self-sufficient and may find the head-of-household role very challenging. As one caregiver

(Jennings 1997, 128) reported: "I had to become the decision-maker—about his treatment, our finances, everything. None of that side-by-side stuff."

Managing medication.   As hospital lengths of stay have decreased and as more home care technology has become available, caregiving at home has taken on, on a small scale, many of the aspects of an intensive care unit (ICU). Caregivers may be providing care unassisted in a situation that requires more clinical skills than are ordinarily expected of lay people (Schumacher et al. 2000), especially in the area of medication management. When the IADL measures were constructed, managing medications was generally fairly simple, because there were few medications to manage. Now, however, the pharmaceutical armamentarium is enormous and complex. Medications are administered not only orally but also by IV, suppository, and nebulizer.

Travis, Bethea, and Winn (2000) interviewed 23 caregivers and organized the 122 medication administration "hassles" they identified into three main categories: scheduling logistics, administration procedures, and safety issues. When multiple medications are prescribed, the caregiver must keep track of each medication and adhere to the scheduling regimen, keep accurate records, and monitor adverse reactions (Juarez and Ferrell 1996). One caregiver in a United Hospital Fund focus group (Levine 1998, 10) said, "He takes up to 45 pills a day, and I make sure he sticks to the right schedule, which is very regimented in terms of taking pills with and without food, and at certain times of the day."

Another problem encountered with medication management is getting refills. Because availability or reimbursement plans may force caregivers to rely on different sources for different medications, they may be unable to refill multiple prescriptions on time (Travis, Bethea, and Winn 2000). To offset costs, caregivers may use various strategies, such as mail order plans and office samples. Sometimes, however, the prescriptions simply go unfilled.

Hassles associated with administration procedures in the study by Travis, Bethea, and Winn were worse among caregivers caring for cognitively impaired relatives. When the care recipient was "having a bad day" it was difficult for the caregiver to get him or her to take medications. Caregivers also reported distress about having to give painful, embarrassing, or noxious medications. A daughter-in-law (quoted in Travis, Bethea, and Winn 2000, M415) described having to give her "very modest" mother-in-law a vaginal suppository as a "nightmare. . . . The first time I gave it to her I felt like I was raping [her]." Safety issues were the third, and most common, caregiver concern. When drugs are to be given at timed intervals, the caregiver may have to get up during the night to administer the medication, and mistakes can easily occur if he or she is not alert. The caregiver can mix up drugs and doses, posing a danger to the care recipient. Caregivers felt that they had to be vigilant constantly and were extremely distressed if they believed that they had failed to notice a side effect or had to take the patient to the Emergency Department.

What the ADL-IADL Measures Miss about Caregiving

Family caregiving encompasses several complex activities embedded in but not formally recognized by ADL-IADL measures. The primary one is providing emotional support (Bakas, Lewis, and Parsons 2001), which is the expression of the caregiver's love and concern and the usual motivation for assuming the caregiving role. Beyond emotional support, depending on the situation, caregivers engage in monitoring and supervising the care recipient's behavior; managing medical equipment and providing skilled nursing care, including managing pain symptoms; managing hired professionals or paraprofessionals; making decisions about treatment and place of care; and acting throughout as the care recipient's agent and advocate. One caregiver (quoted in McLeod 1995, 1) reported, "You're a banker, an emotional confidant, a friend, a medical advocate. . . . You're dealing with medicines, the medical bureaucracy, trying to find housing. You have to have an expertise in more than you can possibly know about—that's why people need help." And it is striking how many caregivers, like Sweeney (2000, 44), describe what they do in terms of multiple, over-lapping roles: "Being the primary caregiver for my brother, I consciously and unconsciously assumed many roles. At various points I felt like a nurse and doctor, counselor and friend, care team manager, and insurance specialist and banker. I was the executor of his estate and had medical and financial powers of attorney. In the end, I found out that the most important thing I could be was just his brother." Family members who are overwhelmed with the tasks of caregiving find it difficult to fulfill this primary obligation—providing the emotional support that only they can give. Nor can they take care of themselves or their other obligations to family, job, and community.

Supervising Behavior

Probably the most extensively described caregiver task not included in the ADL-IADL measures is monitoring and supervising the behavior of patients with dementia (Jansson, Nordberg, and Grafstrom 2001). As care recipients with dementia become increasingly confused and disoriented, caregivers have to be alert to potential dangers to the person and to others. Wandering, hoarding, failing to turn off the stove, combativeness—all these and more take a great deal of caregiver time and energy. Performing all the ADL-IADL tasks—bathing and feeding in particular, but also transportation—becomes more complicated when the care recipient is frightened or hostile.

From a series of Internet conversations among dementia caregivers, Mahoney (2003) developed the concept of caregiver "vigilance," which includes watchful supervision, protective intervening, anticipating, on duty, and being there. Experienced caregivers "developed a type of unique knowledge about factors that calmed, upset, confused, or oriented their relative" (27). Unfortunately, this special knowledge is often ignored or discounted by health care professionals.

Dementia is not the only condition requiring attention to behavior. Traumatic brain injury, stroke, and malignancies may also alter the care recipient's capacity to control impulsive behavior. Furthermore, some medications have behavioral side effects.

Even without physiologic changes, many people do not adapt easily to illness. They may express their anger and frustration at their dependence by lashing out at the caregiver or others in the home. The caregiver also may be angry and frustrated but has to learn to control his or her own behavior in order not to exacerbate the situation.

Managing Medical Needs

High-tech home care.   High-tech home care is a relatively recent phenomenon. Before the 1980s most kinds of medical care involving medical equipment were limited to inpatient settings and delivered and monitored by professional staff. Today high-tech home care is a big business, and almost anything that can be done in an ICU can be done at home, including artificial nutrition and hydration, mechanical ventilation, maintenance of heart function, and infusion therapies. These interventions not only prolong life but also allow the care recipient to remain at home rather than in a hospital or nursing home. Some of the technologies, such as CPAP (continuous positive airway pressure), used to control sleep apnea, may allow family caregivers to sleep through the night, rather than waking up continually to check on their relative's breathing (Smith et al. 1998). Some families find that providing care at home, even under extremely difficult circumstances, is easier than attending to the care recipient in a hospital or nursing home (Moss et al. 1993).

Although high-tech equipment has many benefits, it also presents many challenges to the family caregiver. Caregivers of persons using home ventilation reported feeling "tied" by home medical equipment (Moss et al. 1993; Van Kesteren, Velthuis, and van Leyden 2001), because regular suctioning is required to prevent the patient from choking. Moreover, the caregiver has to be on call to respond to alarms, which indicate too much or too little air. The caregiver may have to get up several times throughout the night to check on the care recipient and adjust the machine.

Feeding is an ADL, but when it entails artificial means, it seems to fit more closely into the category of medical management. In severe cases of dysphagia, unless the care recipient and health care proxy decline it, artificial hydration and nutrition may be introduced. These are high-tech and costly procedures that bear little resemblance to what is normally considered eating or drinking. The simplest form is an intravenous (IV) line, inserted by a needle into the arm, through which the patient receives fluids and medications. Another common method is the insertion of a nasogastric tube through the nose and down the esophagus to the stomach (Dunn 1994). Both of these are generally considered short-term measures and can be discontinued easily if the patient cannot tolerate them or regains the ability to eat and drink.

Gastrostomy is a long-term measure. It involves a permanent opening between the outside surface of the abdominal wall and the skin. A thick liquid containing nutrients is delivered through the opening by a tube or "feeding button" at a computer-determined rate. This procedure is used when the patient has a normally functioning gastrointestinal tract but cannot meet his or her metabolic or nutritional needs through oral feeding.

The most drastic intervention is TPN (total parenteral nutrition), typically used as a last resort for patients for whom feeding through the gastrointestinal tract is impossible, inadequate, or hazardous. These are usually patients with bowel disease or malignancies (Morse and Colatarci 1994). In TPN, nutrition and hydration are supplied through a central venous line. According to Smith (1999, 122), once the "the daily aseptic procedures for initiating TPN" are completed,

> TPN is then slowly infused over 10 to 12 hours due to the high glucose-load in the infusion add-mixture. In addition, 1 hour of slow-

ing or tapering of the infusion rate is needed before the disconnection procedure. Finally, disconnection procedures and insertion site care are required. Infusion pumps and intravenous equipment must be cleaned, supplies ordered, and the subtle but overlapping patient symptoms and treatment side effects monitored.

Although artificial nutrition and hydration can prolong a person's life, administration and monitoring can be complicated processes (Davitt and Kaye 1995). The caregiver must understand how the equipment works and then learn how to maintain sterility during infusion, read the monitors and respond to alarms, and observe the patient's fluid and nutrition balance (Smith et al. 1993). If the original connection site no longer functions properly, a new site will have to be found (Dunn 1994). One caregiver in a September 1997 United Hospital Fund focus group described the fear associated with taking on the responsibility of administering TPN:

> He [her husband] went into the hospital and he had to have a feeding tube put in. They put in the feeding tube. It was very frightening for me. My generation doesn't know from computers and it looked like a monster to me. First of all, I've never seen this before. I've never seen anyone have a feeding tube ever, so I didn't even know what it was all about. The doctor had said to me, "Well, we'll have to put him on a feeding tube." I didn't even know what he was telling me about. I didn't know. I thought maybe it had something to do with— I heard it once that they put feeding tubes in the nose. This is in the stomach. They make some kind of incision and they put a feeding tube in and it's attached to a pouch and the whole thing is attached to a machine and you adjust that according to the rate the doctor explains to you and you have to push buttons and it's a whole thing and I was terrified.
>
> I was shown how to use it in the hospital but I was expected— I mean I'm taking him home from the hospital and even though the nurse from the Medicare is going to come and show me how to use it, it's still my responsibility to do it. And then the nurse in the hospital says before you take him home we're going to show you how

to do it and they show you—1, 2, 3—that's it. Now you did it. Fine. Meanwhile, you go home and agonize over it. Do I make a mistake? What happens, the thing, if it doesn't run, it starts to scream. It beeps. It makes you frightened. It made me terrified. I cursed that machine so it broke twice. He's now on the third machine. I hate that machine. It's funny but it's not funny. It's very sad.

The procedures performed in the home environment are demanding and can be similar to those executed by trained nurses. As cited in Borneman (1998, 28), the family caregiver assumes the role of a "home care manager," charged with identifying and reporting symptoms, providing emotional support, and handling emergencies. The responsibilities of one caregiver left him "fatigued with very little time to sleep, and with almost no time to himself":

Mr. C, 57 years old, was caring for his 56-year-old wife who was slowly dying of lung cancer that had extensively metastasized to the brain. The physiologic problems she experienced were numerous and complex. They included pleural effusion resulting in shortness of breath and requiring the use of oxygen; severe pain necessitating continual infusion of morphine by means of a pump; intermittent excruciating headaches with nausea and vomiting; and seizures. Mrs. C could no longer walk, eat, drink, verbalize her needs, perform her personal ADLs, or recognize family members. . . . Mr. C was the sole caregiver and was constantly at his wife's side, either replacing the nasal canula for oxygen, cleaning her after an episode of vomiting, performing her personal hygiene, emptying the Foley catheter, providing a bedpan, or being with her during a seizure. He also was responsible for administering the boluses of morphine for breakthrough pain and for notifying the nurse when the morphine needed to be replaced. These caregiving activities required him to be with her 24 hours a day.

Wound management is another nursing-level skill. Wounds have to be kept clean and new dressings applied periodically. At sites where catheters and tubes are connected, it is especially important to maintain cleanliness and sterility to prevent infection. A new infection may mean having to return to the hospital or being prescribed antibiotics (i.e., more medication to manage). A caregiver in the Harvard-United Hospital Fund-VNSNY survey (Levine et al. 2000, 15) reported, "[The greatest challenge] is removing the bandage. Actually looking at the skin being eaten up. That's kind of rough, especially when it is someone that you know and love. I just take a deep breath, wrap it up, and then it is covered."

When a person's life depends on home technology, the home environment can be transformed into a hospital-like setting to accommodate such items as a hospital bed, ventilators, monitors, and IV poles. The caregiver's life also must accommodate these reminders of illness, as in this situation: "Her bed is next to his hospital bed so that she can hold his hand as they sleep, and so that she is nearby if his diaper needs changing in the middle of the night" (Fein 1994).

If the care recipient is able to use a wheelchair, then the home, ideally, should be rearranged to make it accessible. But widening doorways, remodeling bathrooms, and installing electric lifts and ramps are expensive renovations and not feasible in many homes and apartments. Some buildings do not have elevators, and the wheelchair-bound or mobility-impaired person is essentially unable to leave without a great deal of assistance.

Pain management.   Controlling pain has only recently received its proper attention in professional arenas, through hospice and palliative care interventions, and yet it is still one of the least well handled aspects of professional medical care. Nevertheless, untrained family caregivers are routinely given the responsibility of managing pain at home. Ferrell (2001, 596) asserts that "family caregivers who have very little information about pharmacology, dosing of medications, and assessing or treating pain are asked to become the 24-hour-a-day care providers." If professionals are poorly prepared to manage pain, then they can hardly prepare family caregivers in this highly emotionally charged task.

Furthermore, Ferrell (2001, 596) says:

> Professional caring is quite different from family caregiving. The professional's task of spending a few minutes with a patient in pain and then to be able to go home at the end of the day is very different from living 24 hours a day, seven days a week for years on end with someone in pain. . . . Professionals think about the problems faced in pain management because of regulatory barriers, such as what it means to deal with the multiple-copy prescriptions or to be concerned about laws that restrict the number of pills that can be prescribed. Yet, regulation also creates a tremendous burden on family caregivers as they become the gatekeepers. . . . Dealing with regulatory barriers from a family perspective means that you must travel farther to get prescriptions refilled, you must go to different pharmacies, and you must take your loved one to multiple doctors to get the necessary medications.

Misinformation and unfounded fears about pain medications often cause family caregivers to undermedicate their relatives. They may believe that pain is meant to be endured, or that too much medication will leave the patient addicted. They typically believe that the care recipient is experiencing a higher level of pain than care recipients themselves report but fail to report these impressions to professionals because they fear pain means the disease is progressing (Juarez and Ferrell 1996). Family caregivers may be unable to distinguish side effects of medications from disease symptoms. And, without expert advice and intervention, they can only suffer along with the patient. One woman in a September 1997 United Hospital Fund focus group bitterly recalled her father's dying: "I asked the doctor whether I should give him more pain medicine. He said, 'Use your own judgment.'" Another described the worst part of caregiving as watching her sister in pain and having to wait for the appointed hour to give her medication.

Managing Paid Caregivers

When caregiving becomes too difficult for the caregiver to manage alone, or when he or she must maintain a job or care for other family members, home health care services may be the only alternative to placing the care recipient in a skilled nursing facility. In the Harvard-United Hospital Fund-VNSNY survey (Levine et al. 2000, 8), only about 15 percent of the caregivers had hired or managed paid help. Those who did not have hired help either said that they could not afford it, the "care recipient did not need it" (although who made that determination was not clear), or the "care recipient did not want strangers in the house."

Although home care services provide assistance with custodial care, transportation, and medical care, their presence does not decrease the amount of informal care provided (Caro and Stern 1995). On the contrary, the presence of paid help presents another managerial responsibility, as "adult children find themselves operating like personnel managers for their ailing parents, having to recruit workers, check references, set wages and supervise" (McLeod 1995).

Some care recipients are eligible for a limited amount of Medicare- or Medicaid-funded home health care. These services will be handled through a certified home health agency, and the home care aide will be supervised by a nurse. However, the nurse may not make a visit while the aide is present, and the aides may not stay long on the case. The family caregiver provides continuity and is ultimately responsible if the aide fails to arrive or if there is a problem.

Some caregivers hire aides privately, through an agency or registry or by word of mouth. Finding and employing qualified and reliable attendants is a challenge for the caregiver. If the care recipient is receiving a minimum number of hours, it is difficult to hire workers, since most attendants prefer full-time assignments. As a consequence, the turnover rate is high, and the care recipient is continually adjusting to new staff. Furthermore, the caregiver can spend considerably more time training, planning logistics, and coordinating schedules (Davitt and Kaye 1995).

Most home health aides are poorly paid and poorly trained. While many are dedicated and competent, and provide excellent care, a few bad experiences can make a family caregiver and care recipient extremely wary. Aides may not come when scheduled, arrive late, let their own family members or friends drop by to visit, or simply stop coming without informing the caregiver.

Aides may not be familiar with disease management. One caregiver (Young 2000, 26–27) said: "I hired a home care agency whose attendants were trained to work with Alzheimer's patients. In the last eight months of 1995, Mother adjusted to seven home attendants. They were caring people, but some of them knew less about the disease than I had learned in that short year."

Aides also may not be familiar with techniques for handling a person. Another caregiver (Cohen 1996, 40) reported: "The first day was definitely worse than doing the job myself. . . . As [my husband] became more and more deadweight, most of them couldn't [lift him]. They'd try. I'd have to show them or help them each day, before they'd realize and just fail to show up. Or not realize, and I'd have to fire them."

Aides may have emotional or behavioral problems that interfere with their doing their job. The same caregiver said: "The scariest was [——]. He'd talk to himself while we were around, and he'd call me by the pet names [my husband] has for me, in what seemed to me a strange, sneering tone." The boundary lines between family and home care attendant are difficult to set and even more difficult to maintain.

Making Decisions and Solving Problems

The family caregiver is often charged with making decisions with and on behalf of the care recipient (Blustein 1993). The care recipient who is capable of making decisions may nonetheless seek emotional support and assistance from the caregiver during the decision-making process. Or, if the care recipient is not capable of making decisions, particularly during medical interventions, the family caregiver must advocate for the person's needs. Decisions may involve simple matters of daily routine and activities, including pain management. Although each decision may seem minor, taken together they determine quality of life for both care recipient and caregiver. Major decisions alter the goals and plan of care.

Deciding where the person is going to live.   In the course of managing another person's health care, the caregiver typically arrives at a point where a decision must be made regarding where that person will live, especially if the caregiver lives in a different area and is essentially managing the care recipient's health by telephone or occasional visits. Moving the person closer will allow him or her to maintain some level of independence. However, the caregiver may find it more manageable to move the person in with him or her, because it will be easier to integrate care tasks into the household (Gaugler, Kane, and Langlois 2000).

Deciding when to move the person to a nursing facility.   Despite the toll of caregiving, the family caregiver may resist moving an elderly or chronically ill relative into a nursing home or assisted living facility. The expense of skilled nursing facilities can be a huge financial burden, particularly if the care recipient is not eligible for Medicaid. In this situation, the caregiver believes that providing care in the home is the only way to control expenses. Furthermore, the caregiver may also believe that the care recipient is better off at home, surrounded by relatives, because interaction and stimulation are vital to that person's well-being. One caregiver (quoted in Fein 1994) prefers to keep her mother at home, "where she is more confident about the care and they can spend more time together, even if her mother doesn't realize it."

Fear of mistreatment in an institution will often cause a caregiver to delay moving the care recipient. One caregiver (quoted in Fein 1994) reported that "he considered a nursing home but had found the expense too great. He also figured he would spend so much time traveling to visit his mother and would worry so much that she was being mistreated that the stress would barely ease."

When, however, the caregiver can no longer cope with the responsibility of in-home care and, furthermore, realizes that the care recipient needs more care than can be provided at home, he or she may choose to place the care recipient in a nursing home. One caregiver (quoted in Zeigler 1990, 17) reflected: "After twenty-two years of marriage, the marriage as I had known it ceased to exist. We became parent and child. . . . After four years of coping alone, I placed my husband in a facility where he has been since. . . . This is a devastating experience."

The care recipient's health may reach a stage where he or she requires around-the-clock care, and the caregiver is physically, emotionally, and mentally spent. Heavy lifting becomes unbearable, and the sophistication of drug management and high-tech home technology becomes too much for one person to manage adequately. And it becomes more difficult to watch the family member deteriorate—he or she no longer seems to be the familiar and loved figure. The caregiver is afraid to leave the home or leave the care recipient in the care of someone else, in the event that something happens. Nevertheless, when the care recipient moves to a nursing home or skilled nursing facility, the caregiver experiences a sense of guilt (Karlin, Bell, and Noah 2001), as if he or she has abandoned the person.

Caregiving does not end with nursing home placement. Frequent visits are imperative, particularly since the individual is not getting the personal attention once received at home. The caregiver also has to continue to monitor the person's behavioral pattern and alert the nursing home staff to illness, lost mobility, or isolation from other residents. If the care recipient is unhappy in the nursing home, then he or she may not eat or take medication unless the caregiver is present. Moreover, if the individual's hygiene and grooming appear to be a problem, the caregiver may have to take on the responsibility of bathing the person and washing clothes.

Deciding to forgo life support.   Deciding against introducing or continuing mechanical means of life support "is a deliberative process involving information from the past, from the present, and from future projections [and] . . . consenting to discontinuation of life support [must feel] intellectually, emotionally, and morally right" to the caregiver (Swigart et al. 1996, 490). Ideally, the family caregiver and the care recipient should prepare advance directives, such as a durable power of attorney for health care, a living will, or the assignment of a health care proxy, and discuss the care recipient's desires in the event he or she is not able to make decisions. Taking such action, however, is often avoided.

Negotiating the Health Care System

Advocacy is necessary because medical care has become increasingly fragmented and complicated. Trying to advocate on behalf of the care recipient can be frustrating to the caregiver, particularly when physicians and other health care professionals fail to keep him or her informed about the care recipient's health. Care partners report frequent problems with their level of participation and communication with providers (vom Eigen et al. 1999). One man (quoted in Levine 1998, 10) reported: "I take care of my boyfriend who has AIDS. . . . When I ask, 'When is the spinal tap going to take place?' the nurses won't tell me. . . . The biggest problem with going to the hospital is that no one acknowledges that I am important to the health care of the patient. I feel as though I am fending for myself and defending my partner."

When seeking an opinion or information from a physician, the caregiver and the care recipient are probably already extremely anxious. They may not be familiar with medical terminology, and the physician may give a diagnosis without translating what it means into "psychosocial terms for the family" (Strong 1997). The physician also may not give the caregiver and care recipient time to process a diagnosis before proceeding to make arrangements for surgical or medical interventions. When a family member was "admitted to an oncology floor for a cancer workup," for example, the caregiver (Rolland 1995, 1, 3) said:

> The physician never asked us how we wanted to handle information. Three days later, when he came into the room, he asked nine of us into the hall, leaving [her] alone. Everything had been said in that moment. The message was "We are now going to talk about diagnosis and prognosis and we're going to do it separate from [her]." It took me three days to realize I was angry. . . . It permanently affected our relationship with the oncologist.

The caregiver and care recipient may also have to battle a managed care organization (MCO) to get coverage for certain medical procedures or durable medical equipment. Despite the treatment value to the care recipient, the MCO may dispute the necessity of the treatment and deny benefits because they feel it is not cost-effective. Some physicians do not want to spend the time in ultimately unproductive hassles; sometimes the MCO will negotiate only with the patient or family caregiver, who is the one least likely to know the right medical terms and justifications.

Even health professionals who become caregivers may find themselves helpless. A social worker (quoted in Alzheimer's Association 2000, 1), for example, reported: "I quickly came to understand how powerless even I . . . was in negotiating decisions concerning [my mother's] medical care."

Consistent with their simplicity and ordinariness, the ADL-IADL measures do not assess the quality of care or the skills necessary to provide the care. Yet many of these tasks do require specialized knowledge and skills unprecedented for lay persons, sophisticated communication abilities, and the ability to reason and exercise judgment. In suggesting a guide to assess family caregiving skills, Schumacher and colleagues (2000, 191) point out that "family caregiving skill has never been formally developed as a concept in nursing." Yet nursing is the medical profession most consistently described as responsible for training family caregivers. Without direction, support, or training, family caregivers continue to do whatever needs to be done in a job that is only sketchily covered by "assisting with ADLs and IADLs."

Appendix

Individualized Shower Care Plan for Mrs. S

Needs identified:
For comfort— has pain particularly in her legs and feet
To be warm
To feel safe

Behavioral symptoms:
Crying, complaints of being cold, in pain
Refusing shower

Goals:
Increase comfort related to transfers and foot and leg pain
Decrease fear and anxiety and increase pleasure
Keep her warm

Equipment:
3–4 bath towels, 2–3 baby washcloths, 1–2 bath blankets, 2 basins, no-rinse soap, mirror or figurine for distraction, pitcher or graduate, baby shampoo, shower chair, child's padded potty seat insert

Suggested approaches:
To increase comfort and warmth

- give routine Tylenol one hour before you begin
- shower before breakfast

- assess her level of discomfort before you begin
- turn on heat lamp in shower room to warm it
- pad shower chair with child potty seat insert
- move her carefully and slowly
- tell her before you touch her esp. her feet; touch legs gently then move legs up and down gently before you begin transfer
- use touch and soothing voice to reassure her you care and understand that she hurts
- position carefully in shower chair if has skin breakdown on coccyx
- use Arjo mechanical lift for transfer; tell her before you lift her; pad the legs of lift sling to decrease pressure; give her teddy bear to hang onto or ask her to count as distraction
- keep her well covered throughout shower, lifting towel to wash area; use basin with wash cloths and no-rinse soap solution instead of water spray; sincerely apologize if she c/o pain, being cold
- try singing hymns with her
- distract her with objects such as a hand mirror, cute figurines, pictures, flowers

To decrease fear and anxiety

- wake her up slowly and gently—keep lights low until awake
- distract her with conversation on favorite topics—her son, her husband (he was a minister), the church, Austria, being a seamstress
- speak clearly and distinctly, making eye contact as much as possible so she can read lips
- explain any misunderstandings she has r/t being HOH (ex. she hears "watch" instead of "wash")
- respond quickly to her complaints of being cold by adding blankets etc.
- clean her up before and after shower while in bed if she is leading BM
- soak feet in basin of water and no-rinse soap
- wash hair last—be sure she is warm and well covered with bath blanket before beginning; wet head with wash cloths; use a small amount of baby shampoo; rinse using small amount of water from small pitcher or graduate, deflecting water from face and ears

Source: Rader J and AL Barrick. 2000. Ways that work: Bathing without a battle. *Alzheimer's Care Quarterly* 1(4):35–9. Reprinted with permission.

References

Abel EK. 1990. Informal care for the disabled elderly: A critique of recent literature. *Research on Aging* 12:139–57.

Allen SM, V Mor, V Raveis, and P Houts. 1993. Measurement of need for assistance with daily activities: Quantifying the influence of gender roles. *Journal of Gerontology* 48:S204–11.

Alzheimer's Association. 2000, Summer. *New York City Chapter Newsletter.*

Anonymous. 2000, January/February. An empty box of matches. *Mainstay: Newsletter of the Well Spouse Foundation* 59:1.

Bakas T, RR Lewis, and JE Parsons. 2001. Caregiving tasks among family caregivers of patients with lung cancer. *Oncology Nursing Forum* 28: 847–54.

Ball AL. 1997, June. Now it's my turn. *Town & Country.*

Blustein J. 1993. The family in medical decisionmaking. *Hastings Center Report* 23(3):6–13.

Borneman T. 1998. Caring for cancer patients at home: The effect on family caregivers. *Home Health Care Management & Practice* 10(4):25–33.

Caro FG and AL Stern. 1995. Balancing formal and informal care: Meeting needs in a resource-constrained program. *Home Health Care Services Quarterly* 15(4):67–81.

Cobb RW and JF Coughlin. 2000. How will we get there from here? Placing transportation on the aging policy agenda. In *Advancing aging policy as the 21st century begins,* ed. FG Caro, R Morris, and JR Norton, 201–10. Binghamton, NY: Haworth Press.

Cohen MD. 1996. *Dirty details: The days and nights of a well spouse.* Philadelphia: Temple University Press.

Council on Scientific Affairs, American Medical Association. 1993. Physicians and family caregivers. *Journal of the American Medical Association* 269: 1282–84.

Davitt JK and LW Kaye. 1995. High-tech home health care: Administrative and staff perspectives. *Home Health Care Services Quarterly* 15(4):49–65.

Doubrava E. 1998, November/December. Letter to the editor. *Mainstay: Newsletter of the Well Spouse Foundation* 53:7.

Drucker B. 1998, November/December. Letter to the editor. *Mainstay: Newsletter of the Well Spouse Foundation* 53:2.

Dunn H. 1994. *Hard choices for loving people: CPR, artificial feeding, comfort measures only, and the elderly patient.* Herndon, VA: A&A.

Fein EB. 1994, December 19. Caring at home, and burning out: Tending for infirm relatives, guardians suffer themselves. *New York Times.*

Ferrell B. 2001. Pain observed: The experience of pain from the family caregiver's perspective. *Clinics in Geriatric Medicine* 17:595–609.

Gaugler JE, RA Kane, and J Langlois. 2000. Assessment of family caregivers of older adults. In *Assessing older persons: Measures, meaning, and practical applications,* ed. RL Kane and RA Kane, 320–59. New York: Oxford University Press.

Iezzoni LI. 2003. *When walking fails: Mobility problems of adults with chronic conditions.* Berkeley and Los Angeles: University of California Press.

Jansson W, G Nordberg, and M Grafstrom. 2001. Patterns of elderly spousal caregiving in dementia care: An observational study. *Journal of Advanced Nursing* 34:804–12.

Jennings K. 1997, July. Unsentimental: When your spouse becomes suddenly, chronically ill: A tough-minded report from the home front. *Self.*

Juarez G and BR Ferrell. 1996. Family and caregiver involvement in pain management. *Clinics in Geriatric Medicine* 12:531–47.

Karlin NJ, PA Bell, and JL Noah. 2001. Long-term consequences of the Alzheimer's caregiver role: A qualitative analysis. *American Journal of Alzheimer's Disease and Other Dementias* 16:177–82.

Katz S, AB Ford, RW Moskowitz, BA Jackson, and MW Jaffe. 1963. Studies of illness in the aged: The index of the ADL, a standardized measure of biological and psychosocial function. *Journal of the American Medical Association* 185:914–19.

Lawton MP and EM Brody. 1969. Assessment of older people: Self-maintaining and instrumental activities of daily living. *Gerontologist* 9:179–86.

Levine C. 1998. *Rough crossings: Family caregivers' odysseys through the health care system.* New York: United Hospital Fund.

Levine C and AN Kuerbis. 2001. Medical supplies and durable medical equipment. In *The best senior living and eldercare options,* ed. JI Connolly and A Lane, 123–41. New York: Connolly Medical.

Levine C, AN Kuerbis, DA Gould, M Navaie-Waliser, PH Feldman, and K Donelan. 2000. *A survey of family caregivers in New York City: Findings and implications for the health care system.* New York: United Hospital Fund.

Mahoney DF. 2003. Vigilance: Evolution and definition for caregivers of family members with Alzheimer's disease. *Journal of Gerontological Nursing* 29(8): 24–30.

Manthrope J and R Watson. 2003. Poorly served? Eating and dementia. *Journal of Advanced Nursing* 41(2):162–69.

Manthrope J, R Watson, and A Stimpson. 2002, November/December. Eating out: Dementia carers' views on the pleasures and pitfalls. *Journal of Dementia*, 26–27.

McLeod BW. 1995, April 3. No place like home. *San Francisco Examiner.*

Mintz SG. 2002. *Love, honor, and value: A family caregiver speaks out about the choices and challenges of caregiving.* Sterling, VA: Capital Books.

Morse JS and SL Colatarci. 1994. The impact of technology. In *A life-span approach to nursing care for individuals with developmental disabilities*, ed. Roth SP and JS Morse, 351–83. Baltimore: Paul H. Brookes.

Moss AH, P Casey, CB Stocking, RP Roos, BR Brooks, and M Siegler. 1993. Home ventilation for amyotrophic lateral sclerosis patients: Outcomes, costs, and patient, family, and physician attitudes. *Neurology* 43:438–43.

Pearson VI. 2000. Assessment of function in older adults. In *Assessing older persons: Measures, meaning, and practical applications*, ed. RL Kane and RA Kane, 17–48. New York: Oxford University Press.

Pisetsky DS. 1998. Doing everything. *Annals of Internal Medicine* 128(10):869–70.

Rader J and AL Barrick. 2000. Ways that work: Bathing without a battle. *Alzheimer's Care Quarterly* 1(4):35–49.

Rolland J. 1995, November/December. Professionals and families can collaborate. *Mainstay: Newsletter of the Well Spouse Foundation* 35:1, 3.

Schindler R. 1996. Normative crises of the very old and their adult children: A personal account. *Journal of Gerontological Social Work* 25(3/4):3–15.

Schumacher KL, BJ Stewart, PG Archbold, MJ Dodd, and SL Dibble. 2000. Family caregiving skill: Development of the concept. *Research in Nursing & Health* 23:191–203.

Sloane PD, J Rader, AL Barrick, B Hoeffer, S Dwyer, D McKenzie, M Lavelle, K Buckwalkter, L Arrington, and T Pruitt. 1995. Bathing persons with dementia. *Gerontologist* 35:672–78.

Smith CE. 1999. Caregiving effectiveness in families managing complex technology at home: Replication of a model. *Nursing Research* 48(3):120–28.

Smith CE, LS Mayer, C Metsker, M Voelker, S Baldwin, RA Whitman, and SK Pingleton. 1998. Continuous positive airway pressure: Patients' and caregivers' learning needs and barriers to use. *Heart & Lung* 27:99–108.

Smith CE, L Moushey, JA Ross, C Gieffer. 1993. Responsibilities and reactions of family caregivers of patients dependent on total parenteral nutrition at home. *Public Health Nursing* 10(2):122–28.

Strong M. 1997. *Mainstay: For the well spouse of the chronically ill*. Northampton, MA: Bradford Books.

Sweeney TJ. 2000. Learning to be a caregiver, trying to be a brother. In *Always on call: When illness turns families into caregivers*, ed. C Levine, 43–52. New York: United Hospital Fund.

Swigart V, C Lidz, V Butterworth, and R Arnold. 1996. Letting go: Family willingness to forgo life support. *Heart & Lung* 25:483–94.

Travis SS, LS Bethea, and P Winn. 2000. Medication administration hassles reported by family caregivers of dependent elderly persons. *Journal of Gerontology* 55A:M412–17.

Van Kesteren RG, B Velthuis, and LW van Leyden. 2001. Psychosocial problems arising from home ventilation. *American Journal of Physical Medicine & Rehabilitation* 80:439–46.

vom Eigen KA, JD Walker, S Edgman-Levitan, PD Cleary, and TL Delbanco. 1999. Care partner experiences with hospital care. *Medical Care* 37:33–38.

Young CA. 2000. First my mother, then my aunt: A caregiver's diary of Alzheimer's disease. In *Always on call: When illness turns families into caregivers*, ed. C Levine, 21–32. New York: United Hospital Fund.

Zeigler EA. 1990, January/February. Reflections of a spouses' group. *Cognitive Rehabilitation*, 14–19.

2

The Work of Caregiving:
What Do ADLs and IADLs Tell Us?

Susan C. Reinhard

SUMMARY

The initial version of the ADL (activities of daily living) measure was developed in the 1950s and published in 1963. It was designed to measure the course of recovery in older adults who had suffered hip fractures and later other diagnoses. The earliest IADL (instrumental activities of daily living) measure, published in 1969, included aspects of independent living, such as shopping, cooking, and managing money. At present there are over 40 different clinical and survey indexes of functional status.

When family caregiver research began in earnest in the 1980s, researchers applied the ADL and IADL scales to caregivers, on the assumption that what caregivers provided was the mirror image of the functional limitations of the care recipient. While this approach has intuitive appeal, it fails to consider many aspects of caregiving. Moreover, the use of ADLs as proxy measures for caregiver activity has been flawed from the beginning, since there is so much measurement error in ADLs even for their intended purpose.

These scales moved into public policy realms in the 1980s. The initial link was the 1982 informal caregiver supplement to the National Long-Term Care Survey of Medicare Beneficiaries. There are practical consequences for care recipients and their family caregivers, such as their use for eligibility for both private and publicly funded benefits for older adults. For example, most long-term care insurance policies use limitations in ADLs as a threshold, tax credit proposals do the same, and states frequently use ADL limitations to define nursing home eligibility under Medicaid.

More refined measures, or entirely new approaches, are needed to describe the work of caregiving more accurately.

A FAMILY MEMBER'S experience in providing care to a relative who needs assistance varies from person to person, from situation to situation, and across time—to name only a few variables. One variable that has received much attention in the research and policy worlds is the care recipient's level of functioning as measured by ADLs and IADLs. This chapter re-examines the historical, conceptual, and practical bases for applying these measures to the family caregiving experience.

A review of the ADL-IADL literature establishes the historical evolution of these measures from clinical research in the 1960s to the larger world of gerontological research during the past three decades. The clearest conceptual link between ADL and IADL measures and the caregiving experience is evident in caregiver burden research. The initial policy link to informal caregivers emerges in the national policy research activities beginning in the early 1980s. This link continues in policies proposed today, more than 30 years later.

Historical Evolution of ADL-IADL Measures

Conceptual and Practical Origins

Although the first published index that included "everyday activities . . . necessary for ordinary living" for "crippled children" came out in 1935 (Sheldon), measures of ADLs for older adults were first developed in the 1950s, when Sidney Katz and colleagues began their research; they published their seminal work (Katz et al. 1963) a decade later. These clinical researchers worked for eight years to develop a measure of graded physical functioning to study results of treatment and prognosis in elders with hip fractures (and later other diagnoses, such as cerebral infarction, multiple sclerosis, and other chronic illnesses). They also viewed the measure as a survey instrument, a rehabilitation teaching aid, and a tool for studying the aging process. Its theoretical basis was primary biological and psychosocial functioning, postulating that the order of functional recovery follows the order of development of primary functions in children "reflecting the adequacy of organized neurological and locomotor response" (914).

The Index of Independence in Activities of Daily Living (Index of ADL) includes six functions that people perform "habitually and universally" (bathing, dressing, toileting, transferring, continence, and feeding). Adequacy in these functions is expressed as a grade ranging from independence in all six functions to dependence in all six functions. Independence is graded as no supervision, direction, or active personal assistance, with some caveats. For example, independence in bathing could mean the person needs assistance with bathing only a single part of the body (such as a disabled extremity). For caregivers, this definition of independence means the person still needs help— regularly and perhaps strenuously, depending on the part, such as lifting a 300-pound husband's paralyzed leg while he "independently" sponge bathes the rest. There is no mention of who gathers the needed equipment for a sponge bath. In other ADL domains, a person who cannot tie his shoes or cut her meat and butter her bread is still considered independent. It is curious why the clinical researchers did not consider assistance with these kinds of daily activity issues of dependency for those who are helping to tie shoes and "set up" meals.

This classic research, which views ADLs in a hierarchy, holds that recovering patients pass through three stages—early recovery of independence in feeding and continence, subsequent recovery of transfer and going to the toilet, and, finally, recovery of independence in bathing and dressing. This order of recovery reflects childhood growth and development. Theoretically, loss of function in the aging process would follow this orderly development in reverse, with the loss of the most complex and least basic preceding the loss of the most basic and least complex. Early loss ADLs (more complex ADLs) would include bathing, dressing, and toileting independently. Late loss ADLs would include transferring (such as bed mobility), continence, and eating (Morris and Morris 1997; Pearson 2000).

Although used as patient-centered measures of functional abilities for rehabilitation purposes, the link to family caregivers is made even in the early work on ADLs. Katz and colleagues (1963, 918) claim that "the patient who is able to bathe and dress himself and transfer independently requires much less assistance from his family or attendants than one who is limited in those spheres." The implication is that the physician should consider using expensive hospital facilities for physical therapy to improve functional status from the patient's perspective, even if the patient shows only low-grade disease activity through clinical indexes—a welcome view from the caregiver's perspective.

Many other functional assessment scales were developed during the 1960s by clinical researchers and practitioners who sought scales best suited for their own purposes. One scale developed during that period stands out because it focuses on functions that were not represented in the ADL scales. Lawton and Brody (1969) offered a measure of eight "instrumental activities of daily living" or IADLs. The IADLs were intended to measure earlier changes in functioning and address the "ceiling effect" of ADLs for community-dwelling elders. That is, many older adults might be independent in all ADLs but unable to function independently in the community because they cannot shop, cook meals, perform housework, do laundry, handle money, manage transportation, use the telephone, or take medications. Three activities (managing money, using the telephone, and taking medication) make up the cognitive portion of the IADL tool. Acknowledging the gender-based division of labor for that period, these researchers noted that shopping, cooking, housekeeping, and doing laundry may be the best means of assessing women's competence in instrumental activities, while men's competency might be better measured through their performance in handling money or using transportation. Ability to use the telephone and take responsibility for one's own medications might be somewhat gender neutral.

The purpose of this IADL measure was to develop a treatment plan (including what services the family might provide), support the casework process, aid in teaching and training helping professionals, and provide information for planning facilities and staffing patterns. Within the social work paradigm that Brody (Lawton and Brody 1969, 184) brought to this work, the IADL measure could be used to help adult children "move toward a more realistic appraisal of their own capacity to provide the care required by their parent." The intent appears to be a more inclusive assessment of the physical and social functioning of community-residing elders who may need assistance, with the goal of better counseling to help family members determine their ability to provide such assistance.

Gerontological Research

During the past three decades, many instruments have been developed to measure functional status. Feinstein, Josephy, and Wells (1986) identify 43 clinical and survey indexes, and Kane and Kane (1981, 2000) provide reviews of many of the most common instruments. ADL-IADL status has become a standard variable in gerontological research. The concept of functional status operationalized by the ability to perform selected personal care and self-maintenance activities has become "the most popular way of describing the unique health status and service needs of the elderly population. . . . Inclusion of measures of ADLs is almost as frequent as inclusion of age, gender, and marital status in studies of older persons" (Rodgers and Miller 1997, 21).

With the proliferation of ADL and IADL instruments, the gerontological research community has been debating the merits of these various approaches. Most of the attention has gone to methodological issues, with little conceptual work evident. The hierarchical model of ADL and IADL activities is one area that has sparked both conceptual and methodological debate.

Briefly stated, the hierarchical model holds that persons who are dependent in ADLs are also dependent in IADLs (Asberg and Sonn 1988). As noted earlier, within the ADL measures, difficulty bathing reflects the least severe level of disability, followed by dressing, toileting, transferring from a bed or chair, continence, and feeding (Katz et al. 1963), although Siu, Reuben, and Hays (1990) found that removing continence from this hierarchy improves the hierarchical scalability. Changes in IADLs measure even earlier changes in functioning (Lawton and Brody 1969). A hierarchical structure within the IADL framework holds that the use of the telephone represents the lowest level of functioning and money management the highest (Pearson 2000). Spector and colleagues (1987) claim that ADL and IADL functions can be combined into a single hierarchical scale. Taken together, these findings support a model of hierarchical relationships demonstrated within and between ADLs and IADLs.

The research literature documents challenges to this model. Even Katz, working with Akpom (1976), revised the Index of ADL to be a less stringent hierarchy of ADL dependency so that the individual's psychological and social factors in caring for one's self could be accommodated. Some researchers argue that a hierarchical aggregation, also known as a Guttman scale, is difficult to construct because decisions need to be made about the hierarchical importance of various functions (Feinstein et al. 1986). As Pearson (2000, 28) asks, "Is incontinence with good mobility worse than inability to feed and dress oneself? . . . These decisions are value laden and not universally accepted." Pearson also notes that the gender bias in the IADL scales "can obscure the actual degree of functional limitations" (35). For example, men may be assessed as dependent in doing laundry because their wives usually perform this activity (Asberg and Sonn 1988), not because they are physically or cognitively unable to wash clothes. Indeed, Spector and Fleishman (1998) found that their 15-item scale that combines ADL and IADL functioning is not strictly hierarchical because inability to use a telephone could constitute an even more severe level of functional decline than inability to perform many of the basic ADLs (Kassner and Jackson 1998). Doty (1998; cited in Kassner and Jackson 1998) found that older persons who had three out of four IADL limits (medication or money management, using the telephone, preparing meals) used about the same number of hours of care as older adults who had three or four limitations in ADLs. Rather than a summary scale based on a hierarchical model of ADL-IADLs, total number of hours of care may be a better indicator of caregiver effort (Kassner and Jackson 1998) or a measure of "types of care" that include both ADLs and IADLs in the "Level of Care Index" (National Alliance for Caregiving and AARP 1997).

Based on these findings, a hierarchical conceptualization of ADLs and IADLs may have negative practical consequences for family caregivers when this paradigm is applied to policy research and policy-making that links the functional status of the person with the disability to implied assistance provided by caregivers. To assume that there is no need to measure IADLs if the older adult is dependent in ADLs is to underreport what caregivers do, since 51 percent of caregivers surveyed by the National Alliance for Caregiving and AARP (1997) report that they help with at least one ADL, but 98 percent of caregivers report that they assist the care recipient with at least one IADL. And the assumption that every item in an ADL or IADL score should have equal weighting in a summary score ignores the contextual issues in caregiving.

One example of a contextual issue is the older adult's "effort, collaboration or support in the effort to perform the tasks in functional indices" (Feinstein, Josephy, and Wells 1986). Helping a person who is cooperative is far different from helping a person who is resisting assistance in bathing or eating. In addition, environmental factors, such as living on the third floor without an elevator, may make it almost impossible for an older adult to shop (Asberg and Sonn 1988), though that person's physical and cognitive functioning might permit independence if he or she moved to a more accessible housing arrangement. The difference is of great significance for family caregivers who have to help with shopping, even if the care recipient is independent in ADLs.

There is still no consensus on the best way to measure ADL limitations (Rodgers and Miller 1997; Zimmer, Rothenberg, and Andresen 1997). There is more consensus on what ADLs to measure, but little agreement on how to measure them (Jette 1994). Refinements include measures of physical functioning beyond IADLs, such as exercise level (Reuben et al. 1990), and caution to use operational measures that are consistent with the purpose of the research. For example, on one hand, Jette (1994) suggests that researchers who are interested in the consequences of ADL impairments for health service use should use scales that rate the difficulty in performing ADLs. On the other hand, the need for assistance in various ADLs is more important in estimating the demand for long-term care insurance (or the need for caregiver support). Measures should also clarify whether "standby assistance" constitutes dependency. As one research team (Kempen, Myers, and Powell 1995) summarized, it is essential to carefully assess all ADL-IADL items for "clinical" or specific individual circumstances, and the practical assumption of a hierarchy should be used mainly for epidemiological research purposes.

Conceptual Link between ADL and IADL Measures and the Caregiving Experience

As the gerontological research on ADLs and IADL measures reached the level of maturity to focus on methodological refinements in the 1980s and 1990s, interest in family caregivers began in earnest (Farran 2001). It was not a far leap to assume that when the care recipient has functional deficits, there is a need for help in meeting ADLs—and that family caregivers provide that help. Rarely articulated in those decades, however, was conceptualization of the relationships among the care recipient's functional deficits, the content of caregiving in terms of help provided, and the consequences or impact of providing help (Montgomery, Gonyea, and Hooyman 1985; Reinhard and Horwitz 1995).

The early research on family caregiving focused on the "burden" that families experience in caring for an ill or disabled family member. In the 1960s studies of discharged persons with mental illness placed in relatives' homes (Grad and Sainsbury 1963; Hoenig and Hamilton 1966), burden was viewed as the negative consequences of providing this care. This work did not relate caregivers' specific responsibilities in assisting with the care recipients' functional deficits (Thompson and Doll 1982; Montgomery, Gonyea, and Hooyman 1985).

As gerontologists built on the burden concept in the 1980s, however, they began to use ADLs as an indicator of care demands and a correlate to a burden construct (see Gaugler, Kane, and Langlois 2000 for a current review of burden instruments). Employing a unidimensional construct of burden, Zarit, Reever, and Bach-Peterson (1980) found no relationship between burden and the care recipient's functioning. However, Montgomery, Gonyea, and Hooyman (1985) made a significant contribution to the conceptualization of burden by distinguishing between objective and subjective dimensions of burden and relating each to the "extent of caregiving" measured as assistance with 21 ADL-IADL activities. Seven types of caregiving emerged to define the "extent" or content of caregiving, with some sets of tasks more confining to caregivers than others. For example, "type 2 tasks" (assisting with bathing, dressing, and nursing care) require that the caregiver be available every day at a specified time. Even more confining are "type 7 tasks," such as assisting with walking, transportation, and errands, which often involve accompanying the care recipient to appointments and "put[s] the caregiver on the care receiver's time schedule" (23). Both sets of tasks were significant predictors of objective burden or disruptions in the caregiver's life and household. The researchers concluded that policies and programs could be designed to arrange for assistance with these confining tasks.

Other researchers used ADLs explicitly but also adapted them to be more sensitive to the caregiving situation. One example emerges from researchers from the same research institute associated with the seminal work on ADLs published by Katz and colleagues (1963)—the Benjamin Rose Institute in Cleveland. Poulshock and Deimling (1984, 230) used ADLs as an independent variable in predicting burden, which they view as a mediating force between the care recipient's impairments and the impact of caregiving on families—caregivers subjectively interpret the "problems that flow from elders' impairments." Conceptualizing ADL functioning as one of two measures of the care recipient's impairment (the other one being a measure of mental functioning), these researchers introduced an interesting adaptation of the classic ADL measures. For each ADL dependency, the caregiver was asked to rate whether or not help with that ADL is tiring, difficult, or upsetting—an ordinal rather than an interval, continuous scale. Again, ADL deficits were significantly related to burden, but in no case did functional impairment and cognitive incapacity explain more than 21 percent of the variance in the sense of burden. Clearly, factors other than impairment in ADLs or cognitive incapacity affect family members' sense of burden. Indeed, these researchers call for a "more complex and reality-oriented perspective on caregiving" (239) to inform research.

Kinney and Stevens (1989, 328) attempt to provide this kind of reality-based perspective in relation to ADLs and IADLs. Rather than rely on classic measures, they developed the Caregiving Hassles Scale for assessing "the minor events comprising the day-to-day experience of caregiving" that annoy, bother, or upset the caregiver of a person with dementia. These hassles include assistance with nine basic ADLs and seven IADLs—as well as hassles with the care recipient's cognitive status and behavior, and hassles with the caregiver's support network. The basic ADLs include items that are not typically seen in ADL scales—such as assisting with health aids (braces, dentures), assisting with exercises and therapy, and giving medications (usually seen as an IADL). The IADL items include extra expenses due to caregiving, picking up after the care recipient, providing daytime supervision, and providing night supervision.

Perhaps the most influential work linking ADLs and IADLs to family caregiving comes from the conceptualization of family caregiving within the stress paradigm (Pearlin et al. 1990, 583). Noting that "research into caregiving has become a flourishing enterprise" because informal caregiving is "a typical experience," these scholars conceptualize the care recipient's need for help with ADLs and IADLs as one of the primary objective stressors (or care demands) that lead to caregiver impact (such as burden, depression, and physical health effects). Basing their work on the "standard" ADL-IADL measures (Katz et al. 1963; Lawton and Brody 1969), Pearlin and colleagues (1990, 587) assume that "the more dependent impaired persons are, the greater is the sheer amount and difficulty of work caregivers must perform for them." They feel that, combined with measures of "problematic behaviors" and the cognitive status of the care recipient, functional measures of "daily dependencies" in functional areas can be used to make inferences about the custodial care needed and the demands and hardships that caregivers encounter. In addition, they also consider it likely that the activities of caregivers in assisting care recipients with these objective assessments of functional impairments "come to symbolize the changes that have overtaken the life and self of the caregiver." As such, these indicators of functional impairment might serve as "indicators of the current demand of caregivers and as benchmarks of transformations that have already occurred and those that are expected."

Noting that the magnitude of the workload alone is not a potent stressor in caring for a person with dementia, but that the resistance on the part of the care recipient results in more stress, Aneshensel,

Pearlin, and Schuler (1993) rely on the stress paradigm of family caregiving. In a later work, Aneshensel and colleagues (1995) document that the course of ADL dependencies parallels that of changes in cognitive impairment. Using ADLs and IADLs as objective primary stressors, Pearlin and colleagues (1990) include the component of "supervising the patient" and "restraining him or her from potentially harmful actions." This activity results in a reorganization of complex family relationships that is by itself stressful, independent of the level of care needed by the care recipient. The constant need for assistance and control leads to feelings of "role overload" when family members feel overwhelmed by responsibilities, and even more significantly "role captivity," in which caregivers are the "unwilling incumbents of social roles"—a secondary stressor. Based on this conceptualization, role captivity leads to role overload and the decision to institutionalize the care recipient with dementia. IADL dependencies, more than ADL dependencies, lead to these feelings of role overload and the decision to institutionalize.

After wide dissemination of this stress paradigm for family caregiving, most caregiving research using community-based samples has drawn on this model (Gaugler, Zarit, and Pearlin 1999). Among the most significant findings of caregiver research is that family members continue "non-technical" support even after institutionalization of their family member (Bowers 1988), and the relationship between the care recipient's functioning and caregiver burden may become nonlinear as care recipients become more impaired (Vitaliano, Young, and Russo 1991).

As caregiving research continues, practical applications to the private and public sectors are evident. Applications in the private sector include the search for tools that may be used to test the efficacy of therapeutic agents for people with Alzheimer's disease. Tools that measure the time spent on caregiving might be linked to the economic impact of Alzheimer's disease. One such tool, the Caregiver Activity Survey (CAS) (Davis et al. 1997; Marin et al. 2000) builds from a base of research that over 50 percent of time spent on caregiving is related to the care recipient's deficits in ADLs and IADLs (Rice et al. 1993). The CAS includes the classic ADL-IADL measures and adds a supervision item since caregivers of people with Alzheimer's disease spend considerable time monitoring wandering behavior and other "potentially dangerous behaviors due to impaired judgement" (Davis et al. 1997, 980). Davis and colleagues also add a communication item because people with Alzheimer's disease repeatedly ask the same questions and need repeated instructions. Indeed, they find the greatest amount of time is spent on supervision and communication. Communication alone accounts for an average of three hours a day. Another perspective employs the concept of "vigilance," the time caregivers spend protecting the care recipient from harm (Mahoney et al. 2003). In the Caregiver Vigilance Scale, caregivers answer four questions, such as "In the case of a family emergency, are you able to leave [name of person] alone, that is, with no one else there?" (Mahoney et al. 2003, 41).

The application of this line of research linking caregivers' time spent supervising and assisting with ADLs for people with Alzheimer's disease was evident in the Tenth Annual Alzheimer's Disease Education Conference, in July 2001, which included a poster session for scientific research. On one of the posters, Janssen Pharmaceutical Products presented findings that a drug known as Galantamine reduced the time caregivers spent supervising and assisting patients with ADL limitations (Lilienfeld and Papadopoulos 2001). The link between ADLs and caregivers has made it to the private sector.

Policy Link to Informal Caregiving

With the broad acceptance of functional measures in the gerontological research community, the public sector policy research community adopted ADL and IADL measures in national survey instruments to estimate the size of the older population with disabilities. The burgeoning interest in family caregiving led to the policy research link between functional measures of older adults and their caregivers in the 1980s.

The National Long-Term Care Survey of Medicare Beneficiaries, first published in 1982, is the major source of nationally representative information about adults aged 65 or older with chronic functional disabilities (Clark 1998). Repeated in 1984, 1989, 1994, and 1999, this survey, from its inception, included functional measures with detailed questions about six ADLs and seven IADLs. The primary purpose of these surveys was to predict disability trends. However, an informal caregiver survey supplement was included in the 1982, 1989, and 1999 versions.

The initial policy link to informal caregivers emerges in these supplements. The instructions to the surveyors define a caregiver as someone who gave unpaid assistance with at least one ADL to the sampled Medicare beneficiary. Because of budget restrictions and the underlying assumption that helping with ADLs is more stressful and time-consuming than helping with IADLs, caregiving was defined in relation to ADLs only (Clark 1993). Hence, the national research protocol began defining caregivers in relation to the care recipient's ADL limitations and implicitly used the hierarchical model of ADLs and IADLs to justify reliance on ADL measures. The survey did, however, ask questions about the kinds of care the caregiver provided, as well as consequences, such as costs and effects on working and mobility.

Other national policy research efforts, such as the National Health Interview's Supplement on Aging (National Center for Health Statistics 1987) and the 1987 National Medical Expenditures Survey (Mathiowetz and Lair 1994) also included ADLs and IADLs (see Weiner et al. 1990 for a summary of 11 national surveys that include functional measures). By the late 1980s, the substantial variability in disability projections arising from these different national surveys became the focus of a federal interagency forum to examine reasons for this variability. Weiner and colleagues (1990) found that differences in the ADL measures used in the different national surveys account for much of the variation in the reported estimates. The surveys differ in whether or not they assess the degree of difficulty in performing each of the ADLs, the assistance received, and the duration of the disability. In addition, respondents interpret the questions in different ways, depending on their culture, language, and education (Linn, Hunter, and Linn 1980). Rodgers and Miller (1997) agree that there is a substantial amount of measurement error in the answers to ADL items, and Jette (1994) notes that scaling methods can produce dramatic differences in prevalence estimates of disability among the elderly. Analyzing data from the 1987 National Medical Expenditure Survey, Mathiowetz and Lair (1994) indicate that demographic, health, and ADL measures are more useful in predicting decline than improvements because of methodological factors—improvements in ADL status may be overestimated in the cross-sectional estimates of ADL limitations. The authors warn that the lack of stability in ADL measures "suggest[s] that difficulties may be encountered in applying these measures in assessment situations for long-term care eligibility" (260).

Given these findings, it would seem that the use of ADLs as a proxy measure for caregiver activity has been flawed from the beginning, since there is so much measurement error in ADLs even for their intended purpose of examining the disabilities of care recipients. If caregivers are defined as helping with at least one ADL and yet there is substantial variation in the answers to ADL items, the definitional assumptions for caregiving in policy research rest on a shaky foundation.

Domains Represented in ADL-IADL Measures

A fundamental question in using ADL-IADL measures to define the work of caregiving is the content of the items or the domains represented. For example, while there is consensus that assistance with bathing is a domain for common caregiver activity, Sloane and colleagues (1995, 678) have provided compelling evidence that bathing "is not simply a mechanical task, but rather a craft requiring complex skills, assessment, and creativity," especially when the care recipient is reluctant (Radar and Barrick 2000). In addition, assistance with the classic domains, such as bathing or shopping, does not appear to reflect the more recent research or the current realities of the everyday life of caregivers. For example, Davis and colleagues (1997) have documented the considerable amount of time that caregivers spend communicating with care recipients who have Alzheimer's disease and ask repetitive questions or need many directions to accomplish simple tasks. Supervising the person to ensure safety related to impaired judgment and wandering is another domain not represented in the common ADL-IADL measures (Davis et al. 1997; Marin et al. 2000). A measure of "being able to be left alone" maps well with hours of care a caregiver provides because the care recipient is not safe to be left alone (K. Maslow, personal communication, July 12, 2001).

Perhaps because the conceptualization of ADLs and IADLs began almost five decades ago, they do not appear to capture the current realities of managing a chronic health problem with acute exacerbations that require intermittent hospitalizations, and with "rough crossings" between home, hospital, and other institutional settings (Levine 1998). Katz and colleagues (1963) in the early 1960s, and Lawton and Brody (1969) in the late 1960s, could not have imagined the use of complex medication regimens and technologies that are commonly used today in the home setting (Travis, Bethea, and Winn 2000). "Assistance with medication administration" today is far different from that task 30 years ago. People are discharged from hospitals after fairly brief stays and are expected to manage multiple prescriptions with serious side effects if not taken properly—side effects that result in confusion, falls, seriously altered body chemistry, and death. They are also expected to manage dressing changes, suctioning equipment, oxygen, feeding tubes, catheters, injections, and intravenous therapy (Mezey 1999; Reinhard, Rosswurm, and Robinson 2000). Because few people who are ill enough to require these complex treatments are well enough to handle them alone, families are often called in to assist. They are asked to do "things that make nursing students tremble" (Reinhard 2001). Yet the management of complex medication schedules, medical treatments, and the use of medical equipment is not part of the generally accepted IADL measures.

Another neglected domain that would not be as evident in the 1960s and 1970s is the increasingly complex and frustrating work of interacting with the formal health care system and social service systems, including application for public assistance (Grant 1996; Jones 1994; Levine 2000; National Alliance for Caregiving and AARP 1997; Vitaliano, Young, and Russo 1991; Vitaliano, Russo, et al. 1991). These activities include negotiating with managed care organizations and insurance companies, seeking public assistance, locating and providing required documentation for the approval and payment of services, seeking and mobilizing equipment and supplies, making appointments, and supervising formal caregivers, such as home health aides. Yet this set of instrumental activities of daily living with illness is not part of IADL measures and therefore not part of the disability estimates for older adults or predictions of the need for family caregiver support.

Uses of ADL and IADL Measures for Policy Purposes

Despite the limitations in using functional measures in policy research, and the lack of attention to the domains represented (or not represented) in these measures, the use of ADL and IADL measures in the policy arena continues to grow, with practical consequences for both care recipients and their family caregivers. Notwithstanding the seriousness of these consequences, little attention has been given to the original assumptions that undergird the use of these functional measures as eligibility criteria for public and private policies and programs, especially for family caregivers.

The evolution of ADLs and IADLs from patient-centered measures of function used for clinical and rehabilitation purposes for the index "patient" to eligibility criteria for policies and programs has been incremental but steady. Using the "valid and reliable" measures that could be scientifically justified in regression formulas, the research community found 20 years ago that deficits in ADLs are significant predictors of admission to a nursing home (Branch and Jette 1982; Hanley et al. 1990), although there is an occasional reference to questions about this predictability. For example, Montgomery and Kosloski (1994) found that ADL limitations had different implications for spouses and adult children. The need for greater assistance with shopping, meal preparation, and clean-up predicted nursing home placement for both spouses and adult children. However, limitations in personal ADLs (bathing, toileting, dressing, and transferring) predicted placement in nursing homes by adult children but not spouses. Deficits in ADLs and IADLs alone do not predict nursing home care. The presence of informal support to assist with these limitations affects the placement decision, and spouses and children act differently.

Functional measures have also been used to predict length of hospital stays and discharge status (Asberg 1987; Branch, Jette, and Evashwick 1981), use of paid home care (Soldo and Manton 1985; Liu, Manton, and Aragon 2000), use of informal help (Kemper 1992), use of physician services (Wan and Odell 1981), and mortality (Manton 1988). Gradually over the past two decades, these "established" links between ADLs and IADLs and the need for health care and long-term care services have provided a justifiable framework for policymakers who want an equitable way to establish eligibility criteria for programs and benefits (Kassner and Jackson 1998) or target benefits for those who need the most home care because they are at the highest risk of nursing home placement (Spector and Kemper 1994). Congressional proposals in the 1990s to expand federal funding of personal care assistance services would have based eligibility primarily or exclusively on ADL limitations in two or three of five basic ADLs (Kennedy 1997). Over the years, policymakers have become more comfortable with considering ADL status a major criterion for determining benefits and establishing new social policies (Rodgers and Miller 1997).

Entering the new millennium, ADL measures have become baseline measures for eligibility for both private and publicly funded benefits for older adults. For example, most private long-term care insurance policies require limitations in at least two ADLs (usually out of six common ADLs) to trigger benefits, and all tax-qualified policies include this requirement (Cohen, Miller, and Weinrobe 2001). Current federal proposals to amend the Internal Revenue Code to allow individuals a deduction for qualified long-term care insurance premiums or a tax credit for caring for individuals with long-term care needs rely on ADLs to define individuals with long-term care needs. These individuals must be unable to perform at least three activities of daily living because of loss of functional capacity; if cognitively impaired, they must require substantial supervision to be protected from threats to safety and be limited in at least one ADL without reminding or cuing assistance.

This is a crucial time to examine the limitations in ADLs as the basis for making families eligible for caregiving programs and benefits. As Silverstein and Parrott (2001) document, 70 percent of Americans support tax credits to caregivers, and 60 percent support employers' provision of time off to caregivers. As federal policy for supporting family caregivers is becoming more popular, the basis for determining how caregivers become eligible for claiming support becomes a serious matter of public policy.

One of the most significant ways that public policy has come to use ADL-IADL measures as eligibility criteria for publicly funded programs is in access to long-term care. Access to long-term care services for the care recipient obviously affects the daily life of the caregiver who often has to fill in the gaps for denied services. States frequently use ADL measures, for example, to determine nursing facility eligibility for the elderly (Snow 1995) because the "fact that they reliably predict nursing home admissions" is firmly implanted in policymakers' minds and therefore offer great appeal (Kennedy 1997). And, since home- and community-based Medicaid waiver programs are often based on substituting home care for nursing home care, ADL measures are also frequently used as gateways for home care paid under Medicaid (O'Keefe 1996, 1999) and such innovative state-funded programs as the Program of All-Inclusive Care for the Elderly (PACE) (Wieland et al. 2000), adult foster care (Folkemer et al. 1996), and personal assistance services (Morris, Caro, and Hansan 1998). Indeed, the policy debate is not about whether to use ADLs but what ADL threshold is appropriate (Kennedy 1997). Furthermore, proponents for some services that have not required criteria for functional limitations are now recommending them (Pynoos et al. 1995).

This eligibility threshold has found its way to programs that are ostensibly designed to support the caregiver of "nursing home eligible" persons. Feinberg and Pilisuk (1999) found in their survey of 15 states' caregiver support programs that 28 of 33 programs use some type of eligibility criteria for the caregiver that relates to the impairment of the care recipient. Thirteen programs stipulate that the care recipient must be in need of "nursing home level of care," or similar language, which often requires an ADL assessment. For example, New York's Expanded In-Home Services to the Elderly program provides respite care for the caregiver, but the care recipient must have a functional impairment in at least one ADL or two IADLs. Rarely is there a requirement for a caregiver assessment. Although eligibility criteria for state-supported services for family caregivers vary substantially among the states (Coleman 2000), the propensity to frame need in "the most rudimentary acts of survival" represented in the care recipient's ADLs (Kennedy 1997) is a problem for caregivers who do more than help with baths and feeding.

Implications

Because it is difficult to establish the needs of persons with disabilities and their family caregivers, reliance on ADL and IADL measures as criteria for entry into programs such as housing, home care, and respite is problematic—"however appealing these pseudomedical markers may be" (Aneshensel et al. 1995, 336). While Novak and Guest (1989) argue that reliable and sensitive measures of burden are needed to evaluate the effect of respite care, adult day care, and homemaker programs, the family caregiving experience is more than ADLs, IADLs, and burden—although they are related in complex ways within a stress paradigm.

If we accept burden as at least a subjective measure of caregiving impact, the care recipient's impairments in ADLs and IADLs explain perhaps 20 percent of the caregiving experience (Poulshock and Deimling 1984)—a respectable finding in social science research. Functional impairments may be "primary stressors" and proxy measures of the content of caregiving (or demands)—what caregivers do to help compensate for the care recipient's declining function. However, as much as 80 percent of the caregiving impact remains unexplained in this framework. That is a lot of variance to be considered rationale for policymaking. Using ADL and IADL measures may feel "fair" to policymakers but may not provide a strong basis for policymaking. The consistent finding that national surveys that use functional measures produce variable results in predicting disability trends suggests that using these measures for policymaking should at least be re-examined.

The suitability of established indexes, particularly in relation to the specificity of the measures and the domains that affect caregivers, is an important area for discussion. Researchers generally seek broad measures with established psychometric properties, and it takes considerable effort to develop and test new measures. Clinicians seek measures that have more specificity and relevance to the client problems they are examining and are generally more open to developing new measures (hence the proliferation of functional measures and burden instruments). For example, Given and colleagues (1992) argue for a common set of measures of reactions to caregiving. In contrast, Vitaliano, Young, and Russo (1991) argue for measures that are more sensitive to specific problems that diverse caregivers face (caregivers of people with dementia versus caregivers of people with other problems) and measures that are more sensitive to changes over time. Others agree that functional indexes should be based on "clinical sensibility" rather than merely the statistical coefficients for reliability and validity; the setting and purpose is crucial, even though it takes time to develop a specific, simple index (Feinstein, Josephy, and Wells 1986).

Policymaking falls between these broad, scientifically justifiable and client-specific perspectives. Policymakers answer to constituents and often develop policies without research justification, or even in contradiction to research findings. The higher the fiscal impact of the proposed policy, the greater the impulse to narrow its scope. In long-term care and caregiving, this narrowing results in targeting efforts that require some justifiable framework. With decades of research to provide some level of comfort for this justification, policymakers continue to turn to functional measures for this targeting.

One approach to addressing the current limits to these functional measures in relation to caregiving may be to refine them to be consistent with a more reality-oriented perspective on caregiving. Adding or redefining domains (particularly supervision, communication, complex nursing care, and health system navigation) may be helpful. Abandoning the hierarchical model of functional measures and making sure that both ADL and IADL questions are asked may also be warranted. Relying on hours of care, regardless of particular functional impairments, might be more appropriate for policymaking, although getting to the number of hours usually requires questions about the kinds of assistance provided.

Another approach might be abandoning functional measures—or other similar quantifiable, "objective" measures—and relying instead on more discretionary methods. Aneshensel and colleagues (1995, 336, 338) argue that public policies for the support of family caregivers need to be based on "unprecedented flexibility" because even impaired elders and caregivers who are at the same stage of their illnesses and their caregiving careers differ substantially in their needs for assistance and support. Policies that require a physician certification or care manager's judgment are consistent with this perspective, although subject to criticisms of fairness.

Conclusion

This chapter provides a starting point for raising questions as thoughtful scholars, policymakers, and advocates re-examine the use of ADLs and IADLs in relation to the work of caregiving and in particular to the use of these measures by state and federal policymakers as rationales for eligibility and targeting purposes in policy development.

References

Aneshensel CS, LI Pearlin, JT Mullan, SH Zarit, and CJ Whitlatch. 1995. *Profiles in caregiving: The unexpected career.* New York: Academic Press.

Aneshensel CS, LI Pearlin, and RH Schuler. 1993. Stress, role captivity, and the cessation of caregiving. *Journal of Health and Social Behavior* 34:54–70.

Asberg KH. 1987. Disability as a predictor of outcome for the elderly in a department of internal medicine. *Scandinavian Journal of Social Medicine* 15: 261–65.

Asberg K and U Sonn. 1988. The cumulative structure of personal and instrumental ADL. *Scandinavian Journal of Rehabilitation Medicine* 21:171–77.

Bowers B. 1988. Family perceptions of care in a nursing home. *Gerontologist* 28:361–68.

Branch LG and AM Jette. 1982. A prospective study of long-term care institutionalization among the aged. *American Journal of Public Health* 72:1372–79.

Branch LG, AM Jette, and C Evashwick. 1981. Toward understanding elders' health services utilization. *Journal of Community Health* 7:80–92.

Clark R. 1993. *The national long-term care surveys (1982, 1984, 1989).* aspe.os. dhhs.gov/daltcp/reports/nltcssum.htm, accessed January 12, 2004.

———. 1998. *An introduction to the national long-term care surveys.* aspe.os. dhhs.gov/daltcp/reports/nltcssu2.htm, accessed January 12, 2004.

Cohen MA, J Miller, and M Weinrobe. 2001. Patterns of informal and formal caregiving among elders with private long-term care insurance. *Gerontologist* 41:180–87.

Coleman B. 2000. *Helping the helpers: State-supported services for family caregivers.* Washington, DC: AARP Public Policy Institute.

Davis KL, DB Marin, R Kane, D Patrick, E Peskind, MA Raskind, and KL Puder. 1997. The caregiver activity survey (CAS): Development and validation of a new measure for caregivers of persons with Alzheimer's disease. *International Journal of Geriatric Psychiatry* 12:978–88.

Farran C. 2001. Family caregiver intervention research: Where have we been? Where are we going? *Journal of Gerontological Nursing* 27(7):38–45.

Feinberg LF and TL Pilisuk. 1999. *Survey of fifteen states' caregiver support programs: Final report.* San Francisco: Family Caregiver Alliance.

Feinstein AR, BR Josephy, and CK Wells. 1986. Scientific and clinical problems in indexes of functional disability. *Annals of Internal Medicine* 105:413–20.

Folkemer D, A Jensen, L Lipson, M Stauffer, and W Fox-Grage. 1996. *Adult foster care for the elderly: A review of state regulatory and funding strategies.* Vols. 1 and 2. Washington, DC: AARP Public Policy Institute.

Gaugler JE, RA Kane, and J Langlois. 2000. Assessment of family caregivers of older adults. In *Assessing older persons: Measures, meaning, and practical applications,* ed. RL Kane and RA Kane, 320–59. New York: Oxford University Press.

Gaugler JE, SH Zarit, and LI Pearlin. 1999. Caregiving and institutionalization: Perceptions of family conflict and sociometric support. *International Journal of Aging and Human Development* 49(1):1–25.

Given CW, B Given, M Stommel, C Collins, S King, and S Franklin. 1992. The caregiver reaction assessment (CRA) for caregivers to persons with chronic physical and mental impairments. *Research in Nursing & Health* 15:271–83.

Grad J and P Sainsbury. 1963. Mental illness and the family. *Lancet* 1:544–47.

Grant JS. 1996. Home care problems experienced by stroke survivors and their family caregivers. *Home Healthcare Nurse* 14:892–902.

Hanley RJ, L Alecxih, JM Weiner, and DL Kennell. 1990. Predicting elderly nursing home admissions: Results from the 1982–1984 National Long-Term Care Survey. *Research on Aging* 12:199–228.

Hoenig J and MW Hamilton. 1966. The schizophrenic patient in the community and his effect on the household. *International Journal of Social Psychology* 12:165–76.

Jette AM. 1994. How measurement techniques influence estimates of disability in older populations. *Social Science and Medicine* 38:937–42.

Jones CJ. 1994. Household activities performed by caregiving women: Results of a daily diary study. *Journal of Gerontological Social Work* 23:109–34.

Kane RL and RA Kane. 1981. *Assessing the elderly: A practical guide to measurement.* New York: Springer.

———, eds. 2000. *Assessing older persons: Measures, meaning, and practical applications.* New York: Oxford University Press.

Kassner E and B Jackson. 1998. *Determining comparable levels of functional disability.* Washington, DC: AARP.

Katz S and A Akpom. 1976. A measure of primary socio-biological functions. *International Journal of Health Services* 6:493–508.

Katz S, AB Ford, RW Moskowitz, BA Jackson, and MW Jaffe. 1963. Studies of illness in the aged: The index of ADL; A standardized measure of biological and psychosocial function. *Journal of the American Medical Association* 185: 914–19.

Kempen GI, AM Myers, and LE Powell. 1995. Hierarchical structure in ADL and IADL: Analytical assumptions and applications for clinicians and researchers. *Journal of Clinical Epidemiology* 48:1299–305.

Kemper P. 1992. The use of formal and informal home care by the disabled. *Health Services Research* 27:421–51.

Kennedy J. 1997, July/August/September. Personal assistance benefits and federal health care reforms: Who is eligible on the basis of ADL assistance criteria? *Journal of Rehabilitation,* 40–45.

Kinney JM and MAP Stevens. 1989. Caregiving hassles scale: Assessing the daily hassles of caring for a family member with dementia. *Gerontologist* 29: 328–32.

Lawton MP and EM Brody. 1969. Assessment of older people: Self-maintaining and instrumental activities of daily living. *Gerontologist* 9:179–86.

Levine C. 1998. *Rough crossings: Family caregivers' odysseys through the health-care system.* New York: United Hospital Fund.

———. 2000. *Always on call: When illness turns families into caregivers.* New York: United Hospital Fund.

Lilienfeld S and G Papadopoulos. 2001, July 15–18. Galantamine alleviates caregiver burden in Alzheimer's disease. Poster presented at the Tenth Annual Alzheimer's Disease Education Conference, Chicago.

Linn MW, KI Hunter, and BS Linn. 1980. Self-assessed health, impairment, and disability in Anglo, black, and Cuban elderly. *Medical Care* 18:282–88.

Liu K, KG Manton, and C Aragon. 2000. *Changes in home care use by older people with disabilities: 1982–1994.* Washington, DC: AARP Public Policy Institute.

Mahoney DF, RN Jones, DW Coon, AB Mendelsohn, LN Gitlin, and M Ory. 2003. The Caregiver Vigilance Scale: Application and validation in the Resources for Enhancing Alzheimer's Caregiver Health (REACH) project. *American Journal of Alzheimer's Disease and Other Dementias* 18(1):39–48.

Manton KG. 1988. A longitudinal study of functional change and mortality in the United States. *Journal of Gerontology* 43:S153–61.

Marin DB, M Dugue, J Schmeidler, J Santoro, J Neugroschl, G Zaklad, A Brickman, E Schnur, J Hoblyn, and KL Davis. 2000. The caregiver activity survey (CAS): Longitudinal validation of an instrument that measures time spent caregiving for individuals with Alzheimer's disease. *International Journal of Geriatric Psychiatry* 15:680–86.

Mathiowetz NA and TJ Lair. 1994. Getting better? Change or error in the measurement of functional limitations. *Journal of Economic and Social Measurement* 20:237–62.

Mezey M. 1999. Bringing the hospital home. *Nursing Counts* 2(3):3.

Montgomery RJV, JG Gonyea, and NR Hooyman. 1985. Caregiving and the experience of subjective and objective burden. *Family Relations* 34:19–26.

Montgomery R and K Kosloski. 1994. A longitudinal analysis of nursing home placement for dependent elders cared for by spouses vs. adult children. *Journal of Gerontology* 49:S62–74.

Morris J and S Morris. 1997. ADL assessment measures for use with frail elders. *Journal of Mental Health and Aging* 3(1):19–45.

Morris R, FG Caro, and JE Hansan. 1998. *Personal assistance: The future of home care.* Baltimore: Johns Hopkins University Press.

National Alliance for Caregiving and AARP. 1997. *Family caregiving in the U.S.: Findings from a national survey.* Bethesda, MD: National Alliance for Caregiving and AARP.

National Center for Health Statistics. 1987. *The supplement on aging to the 1984 National Health Interview Survey.* Vital and Health Statistics ser. 1, no. 21. Washington, DC: U.S. Government Printing Office.

Novak M and C Guest. 1989. Application of a multidimensional caregiver burden inventory. *Gerontologist* 29:798–803.

O'Keefe J. 1996. *Determining the need for long-term care services: An analysis of health and functional eligibility criteria in Medicaid home and community-based waiver programs.* Washington, DC: AARP Public Policy Institute.

———. 1999. *People with dementia: Can they meet Medicaid level of care criteria for admission to nursing homes and home and community-based waiver programs?* Washington, DC: AARP Public Policy Institute.

Pearlin LI, JT Mullan, SJ Semple, and MM Skaff. 1990. Caregiving and the stress process: An overview of concepts and their measures. *Gerontologist* 30: 583–94.

Pearson VI. 2000. Assessment of function in older adults. In *Assessing older persons: Measures, meaning, and practical applications,* ed. RL Kane and RA Kane, 17–48. New York: Oxford University Press.

Poulshock SW and GT Deimling. 1984. Families caring for elders in residence: Issues in the measurement of burden. *Journal of Gerontology* 39:230–39.

Pynoos J, S Reynolds, E Salend, and A Rahman. 1995. *Waiting for federally assisted housing: A study of the needs and experiences of older applicants.* Washington, DC: AARP Public Policy Institute.

Radar J and A Barrick. 2000. Ways that work: Bathing without a battle. *Alzheimer's Care Quarterly* 1(4):35–49.

Reinhard S. 2001. Nursing's role in family caregiver support. In *Caregiving and loss: Family needs, professional responses,* ed. KJ Doka and JD Davidson, 181–90. Washington, DC: Hospice Foundation of America.

Reinhard S and A Horwitz. 1995. Caregiver burden: Differentiating the content and consequences of family caregiving. *Journal of Marriage and the Family* 57:741–50.

Reinhard S, MA Rosswurm, and KM Robinson. 2000. Policy recommendations for family caregiver support. *Journal of Gerontological Nursing* 26(1): 47–49.

Reuben DB, L Laliberte, J Hiris, and V Mor. 1990. A hierarchical exercise scale to measure function at the advanced activities of daily living (AADL) level. *Journal of the American Geriatrics Society* 38:855–61.

Rice D, P Fox, W Max, PA Webber, DA Lindeman, WW Hauck, and E Segura. 1993. The economic burden of Alzheimer's disease care. *Health Affairs* 12(2):164–76.

Rodgers W and B Miller. 1997. A comparative analysis of ADL questions in surveys of older people. *Journal of Gerontology* 52B:21–36.

Sheldon MP. 1935. A physical achievement record for use with crippled children. *Journal of Health Physical Education.*

Silverstein M and TM Parrott. 2001. Attitudes toward government policies that assist informal caregivers. *Research on Aging* 23:349–74.

Siu A, DB Reuben, and RD Hays. 1990. Hierarchical measures of physical function in ambulatory geriatrics. *Journal of the American Geriatrics Society* 38(10):1113–19.

Sloane PD, J Rader, A Barrick, B Hoeffer, S Dwyer, D McKenzie, M Lavelle, K Buckwalter, L Arrington, and T Pruitt. 1995. Bathing persons with dementia. *Gerontologist* 35:672–78.

Snow KI. 1995. *How states determine nursing facility eligibility for the elderly: A national survey.* Washington, DC: AARP Public Policy Institute.

Soldo B and KG Manton. 1985. Health status and service needs of the oldest old: Current patterns and future trends. *Milbank Quarterly* 63:286–323.

Spector WD and JA Fleishman. 1998. Combining activities of daily living with instrumental activities of daily living to measure functional disability. *Journal of Gerontology* 53:S46–S57.

Spector WD, S Katz, JB Murphy, and JP Fulton. 1987. The hierarchical relationship between activities of daily living and instrumental activities of daily living. *Journal of Chronic Diseases* 40:481–89.

Spector WD and P Kemper. 1994. Disability and cognitive impairment criteria: Targeting those who need the most home care. *Gerontologist* 34:640–51.

Thompson E and W Doll. 1982. The burden of families coping with the mentally ill: An invisible crisis. *Family Relations* 31:379–88.

Travis SS, LS Bethea, and P Winn. 2000. Medication administration hassles reported by family caregivers of dependent elderly persons. *Journal of Gerontology* 55(7):M412–17.

Vitaliano PP, J Russo, HM Young, J Becker, and RD Maiuro. 1991. The screen for caregiver burden. *Gerontologist* 31:76–83.

Vitaliano PP, HM Young, and J Russo. 1991. Burden: A review of measures used among caregivers of individuals with dementia. *Gerontologist* 31:67–75.

Wan T and BG Odell. 1981. Factors affecting the use of social and health services for the elderly. *Ageing and Society* 1:95–115.

Weiland D, V Lamb, H Wang, S Sutton, P Eleazer, and J Egbert. 2000. Participants in the Program of All-Inclusive Care for the Elderly (PACE) demonstration: Developing disease-impairment-disability profiles. *Gerontologist* 40:218–27.

Weiner JM, RJ Hanley, R Clark, and JF Van Nostrand. 1990. Measuring the activities of daily living: Comparisons across national surveys. *Journal of Gerontology* 45(6):S229–37.

Zarit SH, KE Reever, and J Bach-Peterson. 1980. Relatives of the impaired elderly: Correlates of feelings of burden. *Gerontologist* 20:649–55.

Zimmer JG, BM Rothenberg, and EM Andresen. 1997. Functional assessment. In *Assessing the health status of older adults*, ed. EM Andresen, BM Rothenberg, and JG Zimmer, 1–40. New York: Springer.

3

Recognizing the Work of Family and Informal Caregivers: The Case for Caregiver Assessment

Lynn Friss Feinberg

SUMMARY

Caregiver assessment is important in research, policy, and practice. Assessments can be used to describe the population being served and changes over time, identify new directions for service and policy development, ensure high quality of care, or examine caregiver outcomes. In clinical settings, assessment may determine eligibility for services and may be a basis for a supportive care plan.

Caregiving assessment began in the 1960s in studies of families of persons with cognitive impairments due to mental illness, developmental disabilities, or traumatic brain injury. In the 1980s gerontologists began to study the care that family members provide to older persons, primarily those with Alzheimer's disease or other dementias.

Relatively little attention has been paid to recognizing family caregivers as clients themselves and to building a uniform, systematic assessment process. This chapter reviews efforts not only in the United States but also in the United Kingdom, where carers have a legal right to an assessment, and in Australia and Canada.

Caregiver assessments generally take one of two approaches:

- a brief part of an overall assessment of the care recipient, addressing the caregiver's own willingness and capacity to provide care; or
- less frequently, a separate screening tool for the caregiver.

Differences in methodology, nomenclature, and specific items and approaches make it virtually impossible to compare instruments. There is no consensus about how to assess family care or what should be included in a comprehensive caregiver assessment tool. Developing such a consensus should be a high priority.

FAMILIES WHO CARE for loved ones with chronic care needs face many challenges, not the least of which is a long-term care system that does not adequately recognize their own needs for specialized, accessible, and accurate information; education and training; decision support; financial help; respite care; emotional support; and a range of other services. Nonetheless, the long-term care system heavily relies on family and informal (i.e., friends, neighbors) caregivers to provide care. Virtually all older persons (about 95 percent) living in noninstitutionalized settings receive at least some assistance from relatives, friends, and neighbors. About two out of three (67 percent) older persons living in the community rely solely on informal help, mainly from wives or adult daughters (Stone 2000). Families have been, and continue to be, both the major "coordinators" and the major "providers" of everyday long-term care (Friss 1993).

In policy and practice, changes in the health care delivery system, including shorter hospital stays, have shifted the cost and responsibility for the care of frail elders and persons with disabilities onto family caregivers (Guberman et al. 2001b; Levine 1998). Family caregivers now require a greater capacity to understand health and medical information, seek out and use a patchwork of community resources, and navigate the increasingly complex, fragmented, and costly health care and home- and community-based service system (Feinberg 2001; Levine 1998). Because of the barriers to receiving high quality health care and support services, some families never even try to get help. They struggle alone, day in and day out, shouldering constant care demands over many years. Often the result includes health and financial problems for themselves as well.

The complexities of caregiving and the varied tasks performed make the case for implementing systematic caregiver assessment as part of long-term care policy and practice. Although policymakers and practitioners increasingly recognize the central role that families play in coordinating and providing long-term care services to frail elders and persons with disabilities, little attention has been paid to systematic assessment of the situation and well-being of the family or informal caregiver to determine what assistance the caregiver may need (Baxter 2000; Feinberg, Whitlatch, and Tucke 2000).

This chapter summarizes the history and background of caregiver assessment, considers why it is important to assess family care, examines public policy related to caregiver assessment in the United States and abroad, highlights examples of existing tools, explores areas of commonalities as well as differences in caregiver assessment instruments, and concludes by offering implications for policy and practice.

History and Background

Origins of Caregiver Assessment

Caregiver assessment originated in the 1960s in the study of families of persons with cognitive impairments due to mental illness, developmental disabilities, or traumatic brain injury (Grad and Sainsbury 1963; Panting and Merry 1972). Similarly, sociologists and social workers have studied intergenerational relationships, family structure, and family care of older persons since the early 1960s (Brody 1966; Shanas 1962; Shanas and Streib 1965). But not until the 1980s did gerontologists begin to study the actual care that family members provide to older persons and the impact of caregiving (Gaugler, Kane, and Langlois 2000). Most of this early work addressed family caregivers of persons with dementing illnesses, such as Alzheimer's disease (Deimling and Bass 1986; George and Gwyther 1986; Rabins, Mace, and Lucas 1982; Zarit, Orr, and Zarit 1985).

A review of the literature suggests that the study of family care in rehabilitation of persons after a traumatic brain injury (TBI) helped forge the principles of systematic, multidimensional assessment of family caregivers (Lezak 1978; Panting and Merry 1972; Schwentor and Brown 1989). Panting and Merry (1972) conducted one of the first published investigations to focus on family outcomes, interviewing family members of 30 male TBI survivors in England. Among their important findings were the reported high level of strain on family members, especially spouses, and the value of providing families with emotional support, information about the disorder, and assistance with care planning over the long term (Kreutzer, Marwitz, and Kepler 1992). Lezak (1978), a pioneer in neuropsychological assessment, has long advocated that families of persons with TBI have their own particular needs and limitations. Before placing the added burden of providing primary care at home on what is often a fragile care system, the family's needs must be assessed, and their needs must be monitored during and following rehabilitation as well.

Schwentor and Brown (1989, 8) also focused on assessment of families with a TBI relative, noting that "rehabilitation professionals are cognizant of the need to include families in the rehabilitation process but may not know how to determine if the family is capable of following through with recommendations and home-based training programs." These clinical researchers suggest that family assessment can determine the capacities of the family and their need for support.

Caregiver assessment has also been studied in specific programs, for example, hospice. As early as 1985, researchers suggested that systematic attention to caregiver needs and plans for family caregiver assistance should be a major component in hospice care, regardless of the structure of the hospice program (Amenta 1985).

In gerontology, most of the literature on assessment has focused on the older person, not the family member or members providing care. In their seminal book on assessment of older persons, Kane and Kane (1981) make no mention of specific tools for assessing family caregivers. The sequel (Kane and Kane 2000), in contrast, includes a chapter (Gaugler, Kane, and Langlois 2000) on assessment of family caregivers, with a review of existing caregiver measures. The authors review 24 measures of caregiving impact, including the method of administration and the psychometric properties of each, if available.

Moving beyond the Concept of Burden

In the early 1980s when gerontological researchers first began to study family caregivers in earnest, they focused on caregivers of persons with dementia. Consumer-based agencies and organizations (e.g., Alzheimer's Association, Family Caregiver Alliance) had begun to raise awareness about the needs of the person with cognitive impairment, as well as the family providing care. Since that time, a consistent body of research has shown that cognitive impairment is more challenging, costly, and stressful than physical impairment for caregiving families (Ory et al. 1999).

Most of the early research focused on the notion of caregiver "burden," generally with respect to dementia caregivers. However, the first mention of the concept of burden in the research literature was put forth by Grad and Sainsbury (1963) in describing the burden felt by family members who cared for mentally ill relatives at home (Vitaliano, Young, and Russo 1991). Caregiver burden is a broad term with numerous definitions and meanings, encompassing the impact that caregiving has on mental health, physical health, other family relationships, employment, and financial problems (Gaugler, Kane, and Langlois 2000; Pearlin et al. 1990).

Beginning in the mid-1980s critical examinations led to a refinement of the concept. For example, George and Gwyther (1986) noted that burden measures cannot be used to compare caregivers with noncaregivers because they are designed to specifically capture caregiving experiences. Thus, they cannot be administered to noncaregiving populations to assess whether family caregivers are worse off than other groups in similar life situations (George and Gwyther 1986). Today, the term *burden* is less commonly used in practice because family caregivers in general have negative associations with it, and the term may not be culturally appropriate with a diverse caregiving population.

In the late 1980s and early 1990s the research community began focusing on the long-term nature and consequences of caregiving, conducting intervention studies and going beyond the single dimension of burden to emphasize multiple dimensions of caregiver impact (Haley 1989; Mittleman et al. 1995; Montgomery and Borgatta 1989; Zarit 1990). Stress process models of caregiving emerged, grounded in the sociological literature on stress (Lawton et al. 1989; Pearlin et al. 1990; Zarit 1990). In virtually all of these studies, the focus has been on caregivers of persons with dementia.

Some measures used scales previously developed in the stress research literature, such as the concept of "mastery," or the personal control that individuals feel they are able to have over forces affecting their lives (Pearlin and Schooler 1978). Meanwhile, other measures were developed to focus on the caregiving situation, such as the concept of "role overload" (the experience of being overwhelmed by care-related tasks and responsibilities), "role captivity" (the sense of being trapped by caregiving), and global measures to assess how confident and competent family members feel in the caregiving role.

Gaugler, Kane, and Langlois (2000, 345) point out that several studies have addressed caregivers' subjective appraisals of (i.e., emotional reactions to) care demands and tasks. According to these researchers, "subjective appraisals are similar to subjective dimensions of burden.

Appraisals are, however, more directly associated with the responsibilities of caregiving and can be both positive and negative."

Only in recent years have the positive aspects of caregiving received attention. Switzer et al. (2000) define measures to examine the positive aspects of caregiving to include indicators of the extent to which caregiving has made the caregiver feel needed, feel more useful, feel good about himself or herself, have more meaning to life, and learn new skills. Lawton et al. (1989) and Kinney and Stephens (1989) developed measures to assess caregiver uplifts and fulfillment in the caregiving role. More recently, Picot, Youngblut, and Zeller (1997) developed a measure to assess the rewards associated with providing care. Little attention, however, has been given to the assessment of caregiving competence, confidence, and mastery in carrying out specific day-to-day tasks associated with caregiving and what help a caregiver might need.

The Emergence of the Strengths and Skills Perspective

In all the helping professions, assessment has largely addressed problems and functional limitations. Since the mid to late 1980s, social work researchers and others have increasingly questioned the negative or "problem"-focused aspect of practice rooted in the medical model and are now emphasizing a strengths and skills perspective to examine how people react to stressful life situations and focus on strengths and capabilities (Saleebey 1992).

Rapp and Chamberlain (1985) first developed the strengths model in the early 1980s for people with severe mental illness. The diagnostic or functional assessment fails "to reveal the meaning of that person's struggle and the strengths that lie hidden in that person's story" (Weick et al. 1989, 350). Tice and Perkins (1996, 33) have proposed that "a strengths perspective with older persons and their families requires social workers to actively engage in relationships that position the clients as experts in their life situations." The strengths perspective is implemented through mutual participation and decision making among the person with disease or disability, the family or informal caregiver, and the practitioner (Fast and Chapin 2000).

Caregiver Needs in Overall Assessment

The focus in caregiver assessment has generally been to incorporate caregivers as part of the care plan for the care recipient, not to include an understanding of the needs of the caregiver as well (Baxter 2000). If information about the caregiver is sought during the client assessment process, it is generally to clarify the degree to which the caregiver can carry out caregiving tasks or the willingness of the caregiver to provide care, rather than to assess the caregiver and his or her own needs and issues (Baxter 2000).

An international review of the literature by a Canadian research team (Guberman et al. 2001b) identified and collected both validated and nonvalidated caregiver assessment tools. None of the validated tools identified was found to address a range of caregiver issues or specify caregivers' service needs. The 57 articles and reports found on caregiver assessment referenced 63 assessment tools. Of these, 34 (54 percent) were general assessments of the care recipient with a section on caregiver needs and 29 (46 percent) focused specifically on the needs and situation of the family caregiver (Fancey and Keefe 1999; Guberman et al. 2001b). The general assessments with a section on caregivers, usually designed to determine the need for home care or support services, focused on the willingness, ability, and capacity of the caregiver to continue providing care and how these impacted on service planning for the care recipient. The perspective in these general assessments was primarily that of the assessor, rather than the caregiver. Although some assessments asked the care recipient about the needs of the caregiver, generally these tools did not ask caregivers to assess their own needs and emotional health or allow the caregivers to provide their perspective of the situation (Fancey and Keefe 1999; Guberman et al. 2001b). In contrast, the caregiver-specific assessment tools reviewed by Fancey and Keefe (1999) all had questions for the caregiver on the tasks carried out for the care recipient in everyday care and the issues related to these tasks.

Why Assess Family Caregivers?

Assessment of family caregivers is important for several reasons, and assessment information is used for different purposes in research, policy, and practice. In research and policy arenas, assessment can be used to describe the population being served and changes over time, identify new directions for service and policy development, evaluate the effectiveness of existing programs or a specific service, ensure high quality care, or examine caregiver outcomes.

In practice settings, caregiver assessment may determine eligibility for caregiver support services and be a basis for a care plan and services to support and strengthen family caregivers. As Fancey and Keefe (1999, 6) observe, assessing the caregiver "is a necessary requirement of an assessment tool in order to provide the practitioner with an understanding of the caregiver's everyday experience, to recognize and validate the work performed by the caregiver, and to plan support services accordingly." Particularly with respect to dementia care, family caregiver needs often differ from the needs of the care recipient. Understanding the role, multiple stressors, and particular situation of the family caregiver is essential to any care plan that is developed for the care recipient (Baxter 2000; Gaugler et al. 2000). Gwyther, Ballard, and Hinman-Smith (1990, 59) suggest that "a baseline caregiver assessment can guide, prioritize and target interventions to overcome barriers to appropriate use of informal and formal help."

Assessment also can be therapeutic in helping the family feel better understood by practitioners and each other (Gwyther, Ballard, and Hinman-Smith 1990) and can help caregivers feel recognized, valued, acknowledged, and more able to continue in their role (Maddock, Kilner, and Isam 1998). Anecdotal reports from California's Caregiver Resource Centers (CRCs)—a statewide program that has been uniformly conducting caregiver assessments since 1988—suggest that the vast majority of family members who care for those with cognitive impairments appreciate the assessment process and view it as an opportunity to express their own needs and have their situation taken seriously. The information collected during the assessment not only helps families with decision making but also acknowledges their strengths and the effectiveness of their care (Ellano 1997). Caregiver assessment helps practitioners to "provide a more systematic, comprehensive and objective service and apply best practice across all levels of staff" (Maddock, Kilner, and Isam 1998, 60). An assessment tool "legitimizes the rights of caregivers to be heard" (Guberman et al. 2001a, 14) and also legitimizes the needs of family caregivers themselves, as distinct from, but related to, those of the care recipient.

Public Policy and Caregiver Assessment

Fundamental to the design of a long-term care system is how client need is to be assessed. Relatively little attention has been paid in the United States or abroad to recognizing family caregivers as "clients" themselves in long-term care and building a uniform, systematic assessment process to address the needs of family and informal caregivers. This section summarizes public policy developments in the United States, the United Kingdom, Canada, and Australia as they relate to caregiver assessment.

In the United States, Congress approved former President Bill Clinton's $125 million request to fund the new National Family Caregiver Support Program (NFCSP) under the Older Americans Act in December 2000. The NFCSP permits states, for the first time, to provide support services to address the needs of family caregivers of older persons. The federal program, in various stages of implementation throughout the United States, is administered locally by Area Agencies on Aging (AAAs) through the provision of services in five categories: information about the availability of support services; assistance in gaining access; education, counseling, and support groups; respite care; and supplemental services (e.g., home modification). In fiscal year 2002, the NFCSP received an appropriation of $141.5 million, a $16.5 million increase from the previous year's funding (U.S. Department of Health and Human Services 2002). While the federal law allows for the provision of distinct services for caregivers, it includes no mandate for caregiver assessment. To date, the federal government has provided relatively little guidance on caregiver assessment issues to states and local AAAs.

Prior to the implementation of the NFCSP, some states established state-funded caregiver support programs with various approaches to assessing the needs of family caregivers. While the majority of state programs apply some form of assessment to determine eligibility or develop the care plan for the care recipient, most publicly funded programs in the United States do not uniformly or systematically assess the needs and situation of the family caregiver (Feinberg 2002). In a study of 33 caregiver support programs in 15 states, few programs looked systematically at the caregiver's own service needs, even though the majority of programs surveyed identified both the family caregiver and the person with disease or disability as "clients" (Feinberg and Pilisuk 1999).

In contrast to that of the United States, policy in the United Kingdom has developed from first giving carers* the statutory "right" to an assessment of their own needs and then moving toward the provision of carer support services. Since the mid-1990s, government policy has called for recognition of carers, improved assessment and support to carers, a clearer focus on service outcomes, and better information to show the effectiveness of services. The Carers (Recognition and Services) Act passed in 1995 entitles a carer to an assessment in conjunction with an assessment of the disabled individual. The

---

*In the United Kingdom, Australia, and the Netherlands, the term *carer* is used to describe what in the United States is called a "caregiver."

subsequent Carers and Disabled Children Act of 2000* expands the mandate of the 1995 law by giving carers the right to an assessment of their own needs, distinct from those of the disabled individual, and gives local agencies powers to provide services to meet identified carer needs (Howard 2001). Local social service authorities that also provide social services conduct carer assessments. Although carers now have a statutory "right" to their own assessment, resources have not been appropriated to assist local authorities in carrying out their new, but unfunded, assessment mandate. Moreover, neither the acts of 1995 and 2000 nor the national policy guidance specifies the way in which an assessment should be done or recommends the use of a uniform carer assessment tool.

The National Strategy for Carers was launched in England in 1999, and a year later £140 million was allocated to the local authorities to provide respite care over three years. In September 2000 the government announced that this Carers Special Grant would be doubled by 2003–4, although no funds were forthcoming specifically for carer assessments (Howard 2001).

Although public policy recognizes carers as "clients" in their own right, local implementation of assessment policy is at very different stages and varies substantially from one locale to another in the United Kingdom. Studies have found that the quality and speed of assessments have been low and fragmentation high between the health and social services systems because each is organized differently (Department of Health 2001b; Holzhausen 1997; Howard 2001; Social Policy Research Unit 2000). Half of all carers in contact with social services were not fully aware that an assessment had taken place, or what its implications were (Arksey, Hepworth, and Quereshi 2000), and, in practice, only 21 percent of carers were assessed in 2000–1 (Department of Health 2001c).

---

*The 2000 act was enacted in England and Wales only, effective April 1, 2001, with proposals to legislate in Scotland and Northern Ireland (Carers UK 2001).

Over the next few years a major shift is expected in the British health and social services systems as they merge into new structures known as "care trusts." Pooled budgets for providing services will become more common as well. Also, a single assessment process has begun to take hold to reduce duplication of effort and better coordinate services for persons with long-term care needs and their carers (A. Montgomery, personal communication, January 3, 2002).

The single assessment process, initially targeted for older people, was introduced in the National Service Framework for Older People in March 2001. Local implementation by health and social care systems began the following year with full implementation targeted for April 2004. As with the Carers Acts, the department does not recommend the use of a single assessment tool or endorse particular assessment scales (Department of Health 2001b, 2002). Rather, each locality is expected to adopt a common approach to assessment that results in a person-centered, standardized, and outcomes-based approach. It remains to be seen how carers will be included in this single assessment process, despite the policy mandate to assess carer needs.

Australia has been active in support of carers for well over a decade. Carer-related initiatives have established enhanced information services and education, a network of state carers associations, and regional carer support and respite programs (Pierce and Nankervis 1998). Policy discussions have addressed the importance of assessing the needs of the family unit in community care. While the notion of carer assessment has generated wide acceptance over the past few years (Maddock, Kilner, and Isam 1998), and researchers have been developing a carer assessment framework to incorporate into the care recipient's assessment and care planning process (Rembicki and O'Connor 2001), no government policy on carer assessment has been put forth.

Although families in Canada, as in the United States, have been asked increasingly to take on more and more home care tasks because of cutbacks in health care services, family caregivers are not officially recognized as clients in the Canadian health and social service system. Family and informal caregivers do not have status within home care policy or within the home care service package; assessments and services are geared only to the care recipient. Researchers have been developing and testing a systematic assessment tool and recommending that in the health care system, family caregiver well-being must be of equal priority to the well-being of the person with disabilities being cared for (Guberman et al. 2001a).

Caregiver Assessment Tools

In their international review of the literature, Fancey and Keefe (1999) found that the development and use of caregiver assessment tools was relatively new in practice settings and that most countries lack nationally based caregiver assessment instruments. This section highlights selected tools and guidance in the United States and abroad, illustrating various approaches and methods to assess family care, and explores several promising directions.*

Tools Developed in the United States

Recently, the American Medical Association (AMA) developed and tested a brief, practical caregiver self-assessment questionnaire to encourage physicians and health practitioners to recognize and support family caregivers. Its 18 short questions appear in a brochure format. It is designed to be given to caregivers in numerous settings, including the physician's office while the caregiver waits for the care recipient to be seen. Beginning with the simple phrase, "How are *you*?" the tool has 16 yes/no questions (e.g., "Had trouble keeping my mind on what I was doing"; "Felt I couldn't leave my relative alone") and two global scales designed to measure emotional and physical distress. The questionnaire was tested on a national sample of caregivers ($N =$

---

*For a comprehensive review of existing caregiver assessment tools, see Fancey and Keefe 1999.

150) and found to be valid and reliable (alpha = .78) (AMA 2001). While data on usage are not available, anecdotal information suggests that physicians who have used the tool in practice generally do so in their waiting rooms, and several residency programs have incorporated the tool as part of geriatric or home care training (J. Schwartzberg, personal communication, January 18, 2002).

Although the United States has no national policy on caregiver assessment, a few state-funded caregiver support programs have developed uniform caregiver assessment tools, using various approaches and procedures. For example, California's caregiver support program uses an assessment that focuses on the needs and situation of the family caregiver. In contrast, Pennsylvania incorporates caregiver information as part of the state's comprehensive assessment instrument, which all publicly funded long-term care programs use to assess consumers in the state. Some states, such as New Jersey, that provide a specific service (i.e., respite) statewide also conduct a caregiver assessment.

In California's Caregiver Resource Center (CRC) System, established by law in 1984 and administered by the California Department of Mental Health, the family or informal caregiver of an adult with cognitive impairment is considered the client of the program, and information is collected from the caregiver's perspective. The initial assessment tool, developed in consultation with Steven Zarit, was implemented statewide in 1988 and has been revised twice. The current version has 103 items (Statewide Resources Consultant 1997) chosen for uniform identification and recording of problem areas to help determine the most appropriate type and mix of services to meet caregiver needs (Friss 1990).

Information obtained at intake by the CRCs is collected on all first-time family callers to describe their general characteristics and delineate their major needs. Additional assessment (and reassessment) data are collected on a subset of family caregivers in need of direct services. In 2000–1, 3,420 California caregivers completed an in-person, in-home assessment, averaging 1.5 hours each. The assessment includes demographic data on the care recipient (e.g., marital status) and the caregiver (e.g., marital status, educational level, employment status); legal, financial, and health insurance information (e.g., powers of attorney, income level, health care payment mechanism); functional level of the care recipient (i.e., activities of daily living [ADLs] and instrumental activities of daily living [IADLs]) and resulting demands on the caregiver (i.e., degree of upset); adaptation of the Revised Memory and Behavior Problems Checklist (Teri et al. 1992); driving status of the care recipient; the caregiver's perception of his or her role and mastery (adapted from Pearlin et al. 1990); the caregiver's physical health status; the caregiver's current help situation, including both informal and formal help; adequacy of social support; the Center for Epidemiological Studies-Depression Scale (CES-D); open-ended questions to elicit the caregiver's view of the situation; and a summary section that includes a care plan.

The Pennsylvania Family Caregiver Support Program, established by law in 1990 and administered by the Pennsylvania Department of Aging, is designed to assist family caregivers of functionally dependent older persons or cognitively impaired adults. Caregiver assessment has been part of the Pennsylvania Department of Aging's Comprehensive Options Assessment Instrument since about 1996. The comprehensive assessment typically occurs in the home with a full reassessment every two years or more frequently if necessary. The family caregiver components of Pennsylvania's assessment tool include informal supports and a caregiver stress interview. The informal supports section is used to "describe the help provided and the suitability of informal helpers to perform or continue to perform the tasks in caring for the consumer" (Pennsylvania Department of Aging 2001). After identifying any informal supports for the consumer (i.e., the care recipient), the assessor evaluates the ability of the primary caregiver to continue in a caregiving role by asking him or her or other resources to identify any limitations or constraints on the primary caregiver (e.g., poor health, employed, not reliable, lacks knowledge or skills). The primary caregiver is asked 15 questions (e.g., current employment status, hours a day providing care, emotional concerns or difficulties). An optional stress interview using a modified version of the Zarit Burden Interview (22 items; responses on a five-point scale from "never" to "nearly always") is included in the assessment tool to indicate the caregiver's emotional state (Bedard et al. 2001; Zarit, Reever, and Bach-Peterson 1980).

The New Jersey Statewide Respite Care Program, enacted in 1988 and administered by the state's Department of Health and Senior Services (1990), provides respite care services for family and informal caregivers of the elderly and functionally impaired persons (age 18 and above). A uniform assessment occurs at the time of application to the program, with a reassessment every six months. The assessment is always conducted in-person, usually in the home. The care recipient and caregiver assessments are typically done at the same time (P. Nearon, personal communication, January 2, 2002). The current version of the caregiver assessment tool, in use since 1990, includes questions on demographics (e.g., ethnicity, employment status), health status and social supports, reasons for requesting respite, types of care tasks performed (e.g., ADLs, IADLs, changing dressing or bandages, medication management, assisting with exercise), and the need for in-home instruction. An in-home caregiver education form may also be completed to document the need for skills training. After the caregiver interview, the assessor rates degree of social participation, positive coping behavior, and mood, based on observations during the interview.

In the United States, work is under way to field test a dementia caregiver risk appraisal form containing 48 items for use in the National Institute on Aging's REACH II initiative, a multi-site intervention study for enhancing Alzheimer's caregiver health. The appraisal form has five domains: education (4 items); safety (9 items); caregiver skills (8 items); social support (7 items); and caregiver self-management of emotional and physical health (20 items) (Schulz et al. 2003). While the tool is being tested for use in a research study, the investigators hope the caregiver instrument will be useful in both research and practice settings (L. Gitlin, personal communication, January 15, 2002).

Tools Developed outside the United States

In the United Kingdom, implementation of the Carers and Disabled Children Act of 2000, giving carers the right to an assessment of their own needs, is still at an early stage. Discovering that great variation exists across England in the implementation of carer assessments, the Department of Health (2001a) produced general guidance on the assessment process and procedures for community assessors and care managers. The policy guidance does not recommend the use of a single assessment tool. Rather, it provides a framework for local authorities to use as they assess carers' needs: encouraging each locality to adopt a common approach to assessment, advising practitioners to address the impact of the caring role on the individual carer and to approach issues from the carer's perspective, focusing on outcomes the carer wants for support in the caring role, and ensuring that the carer's own health and well-being are maintained (Howard 2001).

The guidance offers 14 domains to help practitioners identify, with the carer, the elements to be contained in the assessment, recognizing that not all domains are appropriate for all carers. The domains are carer's role, respite and social life, physical well-being and personal safety, relationships and mental well-being, care of the home, accommodation (e.g., long-distance caregiving), finances, employment, education and training, current practical and emotional support, wider responsibilities (e.g., child care), future caring role, emergencies and alternative relationships, and access to information and advocacy (Department of Health 2001a). The practitioner's guide also emphasizes four outcomes found to be important to carers by the Social Policy Research Unit (2000), University of York: quality of life for the care recipient (e.g., has meaningful activity, maintains dignity), quality of life for the carer (e.g., enjoys good health or well-being, has a life of his or her own, avoids social isolation), recognition and support in the caring role (e.g., can define limits of his or her role; feels skilled, confident, and knowledgeable), and process outcomes or the impacts of the way help is provided (e.g., has a say in the way help is provided, feels valued and respected as an individual).

In Australia, researchers and practitioners have been developing and testing methods to assess family care for a number of years. In 1997, the Royal District Nursing Services of South Australia (RDNS) and the Carers Association of South Australia undertook a one-year project with 196 carers to develop, test, and evaluate a carer needs assessment tool. Introducing carer assessment at RDNS was seen as a way to formalize existing practice and identify more reliable information with which to assist carers. The study findings suggest that carer assessment provides strong benefits for carers, care recipients, and service providers (Maddock, Kilner, and Isam 1998).

Based on the study results, the assessment tool was revised for use with all carers of RDNS clients. The resulting Carer Needs Assessment, currently in use, builds on a literature review and work done in the United Kingdom and includes six domains: health status, types of care tasks performed (i.e., ADLs and IADLs) and need for caregiver assistance or training, impact of caregiving using the 13-item Caregiver Strain Index (Robinson 1983), social support, home environment of caring (e.g., home modifications or equipment needed), and knowledge of disease or disorder and situation and identification of priority needs.

Carers Victoria, a grassroots organization that has carers as its primary client, played a major role in the late 1990s in guiding the development of new state and Commonwealth regional carer services.

However, each of the nine regional centers in Australia uses a different assessment tool to meet its agency's requirements. Staff at Carers Victoria do not currently use or endorse any particular assessment tool, although they have reviewed several tools used in practice settings (A. Muldowney, personal communication, January 8, 2002).

Another recent carer assessment project in Australia involves the development and testing of a brief carer screening tool for use by community workers in southern Australia to assess carer needs. The framework for development builds on the partnership approach to assessment proposed by Nolan, Grant, and Keady (1996), which aims to incorporate the carer's opinions, preferences, expertise, and strategies into the care recipient's assessment and care planning process, as appropriate (Rembicki and O'Connor 2001). This assessment project is part of a movement in Australia to transform the care planning process from addressing the needs of the care recipient only to addressing the combined needs of the care recipient and the caregiver (Rembicki, Penhall, and O'Connor 2001). The screening tool is intended to be part of the assessment of the care recipient and used to identify carers who are at risk and require further assessment and support from service providers (Rembicki and O'Connor 2001).

The 1999 Canadian National Caregiver Assessment Tool Project created the first appropriate tool for assessing caregivers' needs in Canada. The project goal was to evaluate the context, situation, and needs of caregivers, considered to be "essential partners" of the health care and social service system in the care of adults with disabilities (Guberman et al. 2001a). Two tools were developed and tested.

The first tool, the Caregiver Risk Screen, has two parts: part 1 collects demographic characteristics and the context of the caregiving situation; part 2 assesses the impact of the caregiving situation on the caregiver. Based on telephone interviews of 76 caregivers, the screening tool proved to be highly valid, reliable (alpha = .88), and relatively simple and quick to use, taking about 14 minutes (Guberman et al. 2001b).

The second tool, Caregiver Assessment, collects information from the caregiver's point of view, identifying key areas of difficulty and the types of services or support needed by the caregiver. It covers eight domains, with sections on demographic characteristics of both the caregiver and care recipient, caregiving tasks, relationships with formal service providers, housing, multiple responsibilities (e.g., employment, child care), financial costs, personal health (physical and emotional), relationships (with the care recipient and other family), planning issues (crises and future planning), open-ended questions to elicit the views of the caregiver, and a summary section to identify key areas of need. This comprehensive tool was tested on 168 caregivers and, on average, took 1.5 hours to complete. The investigators suggest that further testing of the tool is warranted because a few areas reported less agreement than desired. They also recommend further testing on family members caring for persons under age 65 without dementia, since this population was underrepresented in the study (Guberman et al. 2001b).

Guberman and colleagues hope to develop a systematic implementation study of their caregiver assessment tool throughout Canada (N. Guberman, personal communication, January 9, 2002). Currently, about ten home care programs in one region of Quebec are using the screening tool, and two pilot respite projects in Quebec home care agencies are using the more comprehensive assessment tool.

No separate assessment of carers exists in the Netherlands. Rather, the comprehensive assessment process of the care recipient includes a section on the carer. Questions focus on carer tasks, with a list of 17 items (e.g., feeding, providing care at night, helping the care recipient in and out of bed), and how often the carer does these tasks. The tool also asks how many hours a carer is available to help the care recipient and what kinds of assistance would be helpful to the carer (e.g., domestic or personal care help, instructions, respite, emotional support by other carers or by a professional) (M. Pijl, personal communication, November 26, 2001).

What Elements of Caregiver Assessment Tools Are Common? Different? What's Missing?

Consensus does not yet exist on a common set of measures or methods for caregiver assessments. Nevertheless, some commonalities exist between countries and within countries on type and use of caregiver assessment tools. Caregiver assessment tools generally reflect a recognition that caregiving is complex, with multiple components, and typically use a combination of caregiver-specific (e.g., burden) and generic measures (e.g., health status). Most tools assess the type and frequency of help the caregiver provides to the care recipient in carrying out ADLs and IADLs, other areas of responsibility (e.g., employment) or personal health that may be barriers to care, and caregiver burden and the emotional reactions to giving care. Caregiver assessments typically collect basic demographic information about both the care recipient and the caregiver (e.g., ethnicity, living arrangement) to understand the caregiving context and describe the characteristics of the population served. In addition, most caregiver assessments are conducted in-person, usually in the home. In their international review, Fancey and Keefe (1999) identified six common elements found in caregiver assessment tools: type and frequency of current care provision, the caregiver's ability to continue with care, additional responsibilities or stressors affecting care provision, informal support, formal services required, and the caregiver's overall health status.

Existing caregiver assessment tools show important differences, too. To date, there has been little focus on standardization, whether in the development or use of a caregiver assessment tool or the measurement and interpretation of the outcomes of assessment. In some countries, each local program uses a different tool to meet its agency requirements.

In practice, caregiver assessments generally take one of two approaches. Typically, they are part of overall home- and community-based care assessments of the care recipient, with a brief section addressing the type and frequency of help provided to the care recipient and the willingness of the family member to continue in the caring role. These tools focus on the needs of the care recipient, not the caregiver (Fancey and Keefe 1999; Guberman et al. 2001b). Less common are distinct caregiver screening tools or more comprehensive assessment instruments that primarily or exclusively address the caregiver's needs and situation, including an understanding of the social support available to the family caregiver.

Nomenclature to describe domains, methodological issues, and specific items and approaches vary greatly, making it virtually impossible to compare across instruments. Existing caregiver assessment tools differ from program to program in purpose, target population (e.g., age or disease-specific), design, method of administration, application (i.e., depending on the resources, knowledge, and skills of the assessor), analysis, and use of data collected. There is substantial variation in how a question is asked or measured in a particular area (e.g., ADLs and IADLs, burden) and the degree to which the assessment process actually addresses issues from the caregiver's perspective. The types of instrument vary from brief screening tools with single-item questions (e.g., "Overall, how burdened do you feel in caring for your relative?") to domain-specific instruments that ask multiple questions about a particular aspect of caregiving.

Some, but not all tools, assess the caregiver's need for information about specific caregiving tasks (e.g., on medication management, on use of the Internet). Several tools address financial and legal information (e.g., out-of-pocket costs of caregiving and financial strain; emergencies and alternative contacts if the caregiver becomes ill; knowledge and use of advance directives, conservatorships, guardianships, and other legal planning tools). Still others include questions about housing and the home environment.

Many measures used in caregiver assessments were developed for research studies, with small, primarily white, middle-class samples, and are now being used in various forms and formats by a range of practitioners to assess caregiver needs (Gaugler, Kane, and Langlois 2000). Little information is available about the extent to which existing measures or assessment tools have been translated from English into other languages to administer to an increasingly diverse caregiving population.

Five important areas of caregiver assessment are still neglected: the actual tasks performed by family caregivers beyond personal care functions (i.e., ADLs and IADLs), the quality of care provided, the skills necessary to provide the care, values, and preferences of the care recipient and the caregiver, and the positive aspects of caregiving. Family caregiving tasks can range from seeking out information about a disease or disorder on the Internet or calling disease-specific organizations; doing personal care (e.g., bathing, feeding); carrying out medical tasks (e.g., administering medications, giving injections); using medical equipment; providing emotional support; accessing, coordinating, and utilizing health care and social services; hiring and managing in-home help; making decisions about care options and living arrangements; and keeping other family members and friends informed about the care recipient's condition and the caregiver's needs. Tools to measure the range of tasks and specific caregiving skills (e.g., communication strategies; behavior management; filling out forms; comfort in making decisions, coordinating care, supervising workers in the home) are underdeveloped (see Chapters 1 and 2). Similarly, the quality of care provided, mastery of specific tasks, or need for caregiver training and education to increase skills and self-confidence are rarely addressed. Families need better training about the management of long-term care, as well as training in how to be an effective caregiver without burning out (Stone 2000).

Most instruments that probe values and preferences have been developed for research purposes, typically focusing on end-of-life issues, rather than everyday care (e.g., accepts restrictions in order to be safe, has personal privacy, maintains dignity, is part of family celebrations). The assessment of values and care preferences and resulting discussions about decision making are, practically speaking, difficult and challenging for families to undertake (Feinberg, Whitlatch, and Tucke 2000). Nevertheless, caregiving requires an understanding of one's own values and preferences, as well as an understanding of what the care recipient values in life. Little attention has been paid to assessing care recipient's values and preferences regarding care issues (Kane 2000b) or to understanding the congruence between the values and preferences of the care recipient and the needs and practices of the caregiver (Feinberg, Whitlatch, and Tucke 2000). Recent research suggests that family caregivers of persons with cognitive impairment generally underestimate how important certain values and preferences are to the care recipient (Feinberg and Whitlatch 2001, 2002).

Finally, relatively little attention has been paid to the positive aspects of caregiving (e.g., feeling more useful, feeling needed, feeling good about oneself, finding more meaning in life) and to the caregiver's existing or potential strengths, resources, or capabilities. Examples of a strengths assessment may include identifying potential personal and environmental strengths, skills, and resources and asking about how a family caregiver has coped with challenges in the past, what the caregiver wants and needs, and what is going well for the caregiver (Fast and Chapin 2000; Tice and Perkins 1996). Including a strengths and skills inventory as part of a comprehensive caregiver assessment process, as well as incorporating both the caregiver's and care recipient's values and preferences for daily care, is likely to enhance the family's decision-making skills and improve caregiver well-being (Feinberg, Whitlatch, and Tucke 2000; Kane and Degenholtz 1997).

Implications for Policy and Practice

Great variation exists in the United States and in many other countries in the use of caregiver assessment tools, as well as the process, methods, and procedures employed. With the exception of the United

Kingdom, no country has adopted public policy to give family and informal caregivers the right to an assessment of their own needs. Even in the United Kingdom, however, there has been little focus on the development or use of a standardized caregiver assessment tool to ensure that information is systematically collected across the country to determine eligibility for support services. In the United Kingdom, through the local authorities, and in the United States, through the network of home and community-based services, agencies differ widely in their approaches to caregiver assessment.

A critical challenge in the United States and abroad is creating greater equity in access to caregiver assessment. Because of the high degree of decentralization in the United States under the implementation of the NFCSP and in other countries (e.g., the United Kingdom) there are important equity questions about the degree to which family and informal caregivers have access to an assessment and support services to meet their needs.

It is crucial in an assessment to understand the care recipient's functional and psychosocial needs and the family caregiver's competence and coping capacity, as well as his or her own psychosocial needs. Therefore, a reconceptualization is needed in long-term care policy and practice, from solely viewing the care recipient as "client" to a family systems perspective, whereby the family caregiver and other family or friends are considered part of the "client system." Systems theory suggests a broad definition of family as a social system comprising a number of people united by emotional ties and by some form of regular interaction (Buckley 1967).

Developing a standardized, comprehensive caregiver assessment tool for use in practice settings is daunting in and of itself. Even if a uniform tool is adopted, however, implementing a systematic process will likely be even more challenging. As Kane (2000a, 519) so aptly observes, "It is easier for a program to settle on an assessment tool than to find a way to use it consistently over time and across assessors." A

caregiver assessment tool will be only as good as the training provided to assessors in the purpose and use of the tool.

References

Amenta MO. 1985. Hospice in the U.S.: Multiple and varied programs. *Nursing
Clinics in North America* 20:26–79.

American Medical Association (AMA). 2001. *Caregiver health: Self-assessment
questionnaires, resources for physicians.* Chicago: American Medical Association.

Arksey H, D Hepworth, and H Quereshi. 2000. *Carers' needs and the Carers Act:
An evaluation of the process and outcomes of assessment.* York, Eng.: Social
Policy Research Unit, University of York.

Baxter EC. 2000. Caregiver assessment: Learn about the caregiver, distinct from
the person with dementia. *Alzheimer's Care Quarterly* 1(3):62–70.

Bedard M, DW Molloy, L Squire, S Dubois, JA Lever, and M McDonnell. 2001.
The Zarit Burden Interview: A new short version and screening version.
Gerontologist 41:652–57.

Brody EM. 1966. The aging family. *Gerontologist* 6:201–6.

Buckley W. 1967. *Sociology and modern systems theory.* Englewood Cliffs, NJ:
Prentice-Hall.

Carers UK. 2001. *Carers and their rights under the Carers Act of 1995 and Carers
and Disabled Children Act of 2000.* London: Carers UK, Training Unit.

Deimling G and D Bass. 1986. Symptoms of mental impairment among elderly
adults and their effects on family caregivers. *Journal of Gerontology* 41:778–84.

U.K. Department of Health. 2001a, March. *A practitioner's guide to carers' assessments under the Carers and Disabled Children Act of 2000.* www.carers.gov/
uk/pdfs/practitionersguide.pdf, accessed August 15, 2002.

———. 2001b, August. *The single assessment process: Consultation papers and
process.* www.doh.gov.uk/scg/sap, accessed August 15, 2002.

———. 2001c, October. *Social services performance assessment framework indicators 2000–2001.* London: Department of Health.

———. 2002. *Single assessment process: Assessment tools and scales.* www.doh.
gov.uk/scg/sap/toolsandscales/index.htm, accessed December 30, 2003.

Ellano C. 1997, December. *California Caregiver Resource Center assessment tool
training: Presentation to clinical staff.* San Francisco.

Fancey P and JM Keefe. 1999, August. *Development of screening and assessment tools for family caregivers. Phase I. Report on review of non-validated tools.* Nova Scotia: Mount St. Vincent University.

Fast B and R Chapin. 2000. *Strengths-based care management for older adults.* Baltimore: Health Professions Press.

Feinberg LF. 2001. *Systems development for family caregiver support services.* U.S. Administration on Aging CareNet ListServ. www.aoa.gov/prof/ aoaprog/caregiver/careprof/progguidance/background/program_issues/ fin-feinberg.pdf, accessed January 12, 2004.

———. 2002. *The state of the art: Caregiver assessment in practice settings.* San Francisco: Family Caregiver Alliance.

Feinberg LF and TL Pilisuk. 1999. *Survey of fifteen states' caregiver support programs: Final report.* San Francisco: Family Caregiver Alliance.

Feinberg LF and CJ Whitlatch. 2001. Are persons with cognitive impairment able to state consistent choices? *Gerontologist* 41:374–82.

———. 2002. Everyday decision making for persons with cognitive impairment and their family caregivers. *American Journal of Alzheimer's Disease and Other Dementias* 7:237–44

Feinberg LF, CJ Whitlatch, and S Tucke. 2000. *Making hard choices: Respecting both voices.* Final Report to the Robert Wood Johnson Foundation. San Francisco: Family Caregiver Alliance.

Friss L. 1990. A model state-level approach to family survival for caregivers of brain-impaired adults. *Gerontologist* 30:121–25.

———. 1993. Family caregivers as case managers: A statewide model for enhancing consumer choice. *Journal of Case Management* 2:53–58.

Gaugler JE, RA Kane, and J Langlois. 2000. Assessment of family caregivers of older adults. In *Assessing older persons: Measures, meaning, and practical applications,* ed. RL Kane and RA Kane, 320–59. New York: Oxford University Press.

George LE and LP Gwyther. 1986. Caregiver well-being: A multidimensional examination of family caregivers of demented adults. *Gerontologist* 26: 253–59.

Grad J and P Sainsbury. 1963. Mental illness and the family. *Lancet* 1:544–47.

Guberman N, J Keefe, P Fancey, D Nahmiash, and L Barylak. 2001a. *Assessment tools Serving the needs of caregivers: A document to better understand the importance of assessing caregivers' needs.* Montreal: School of Social Work, University of Quebec at Montreal.

————. 2001b. *Development of screening and assessment tools for family care-givers: Final report*. Montreal: School of Social Work, University of Quebec at Montreal.

Gwyther LB, EL Ballard, and EA Hinman-Smith. 1990. *Overcoming barriers to appropriate service use: Effective individualized strategies for Alzheimer's care*. Durham, NC: Center for the Study of Aging and Human Development.

Haley W. 1989. Group intervention for dementia caregivers: A longitudinal per-spective. *Gerontologist* 29:478–80.

Holzhausen E. 1997. *In on the act? Social services' experience of the first year of the Carers Act*. London: Carers UK.

Howard M. 2001. *Paying the price: Carers, poverty, and social exclusion*. London: Child Poverty Action Group.

Kane RA. 2000a. Accomplishments, problems, trends, and future challenges. In *Assessing older persons: Measures, meaning, and practical applications*, ed. RL Kane and RA Kane, 519–29. New York: Oxford University Press.

————. 2000b. Values and preferences. In *Assessing older persons: Measures, meaning, and practical applications*, ed. RL Kane and RA Kane, 237–60. New York: Oxford University Press.

Kane RA and H Degenholtz. 1997. Assessing values and preferences: Should we, can we? *Generations* 21:19–24.

Kane RA and RL Kane. 1981. *Assessing the elderly: A practical guide to measure-ment*. New York: Springer.

————, eds. 2000. *Assessing older persons: Measures, meaning, and practical ap-plications*. New York: Oxford University Press.

Kinney J and MAP Stephens. 1989. Hassles and uplifts of giving care to a fam-ily member with dementia. *Psychology and Aging* 4:402–18.

Kreutzer JS, JH Marwitz, and K Kepler. 1992. Traumatic brain injury: Family response and outcome. *Archives of Physical Medicine and Rehabilitation* 73:771–78.

Lawton MP, MH Kleban, M Moss, M Rovine, and A Glicksman. 1989. Measur-ing caregiving appraisal. *Journal of Gerontology* 44:P61–P71.

Levine C. 1998. *Rough crossings: Family caregivers' odysseys through the health care system*. New York: United Hospital Fund.

Lezak M. 1978. Living with the characteristically altered brain-injured patient. *Journal of Clinical Psychiatry* 39:592–98.

Maddock A, D Kilner, and C Isam. 1998, September. *Carer needs assessment trial*. Adelaide: Royal District Nursing Service of South Australia.

Mittleman MS, SH Ferris, E Shulman, G Steinberg, A Ambinder, JA Mackell, and J Cohen. 1995. A comprehensive support program: Effect on depression in spouse caregivers of Alzheimer's disease patients. *Gerontologist* 35: 792–802.

Montgomery RJV and EF Borgatta. 1989. The effect of alternative support strategies on family caregivers. *Gerontologist* 29:457–64.

New Jersey Department of Health and Senior Services. 1990. *Statewide respite program: Caregiver assessment.* Trenton: New Jersey Department of Health and Senior Services.

Nolan M, G Grant, and J Keady. 1996. *Understanding family care.* Birmingham, Eng.: Open University Press.

Ory MG, RR Hoffman, JL Yee, S Tennstedt, and R Schulz. 1999. Prevalence and impact of caregiving: A detailed comparison between dementia and non-dementia caregivers. *Gerontologist* 39:177–85.

Panting A and PH Merry. 1972. The long-term rehabilitation of severe head injuries with particular reference to the need for social and medical support for the patient's family. *Rehabilitation* 28:33–37.

Pearlin LI, JT Mullan, SJ Semple, and MM Skaff. 1990. Caregiving and the stress process: An overview of concepts and their measures. *Gerontologist* 30: 583–94.

Pearlin LI and C Schooler. 1978. The structure of coping. *Journal of Health and Social Behavior* 19:2–21.

Pennsylvania Department of Aging. 2001. *Pennsylvania caregiver assessment forms and instructions.* www.aoa.gov/prof/aoaprog/caregiver/careprof/progguidance/resources/PA-CGAssessmentFormsandInstructions.pdf, accessed January 12, 2004.

Picot SJF, J Youngblut, and R Zeller. 1997. Development and testing of a measure of perceived rewards in adults. *Journal of Nursing Measurement* 5:33–52.

Pierce G and J Nankervis. 1998. *Putting carers in the picture: Improving the focus on carer needs in aged care assessments.* Melbourne: Carers Association Victoria.

Rabins P, N Mace, and M Lucas. 1982. The impact of dementia on the family. *Journal of the American Medical Association* 248:333–35.

Rapp C and R Chamberlain. 1985. Case management services to the chronically mentally ill. *Social Work* 30:417–22.

Rembicki D and R O'Connor. 2001, July. Development of a carer screening tool. Paper presented at the 17th Congress of the International Association of Gerontology, World Congress of Gerontology, Vancouver.

Rembicki D, R Penhall, and R O'Connor. 2001. *Development of a carer risk screen: Interim report of the Carer Assessment Project.* Eastern Domiciliary Care Services, Adelaide, South Australia.

Robinson BC. 1983. Validation of a caregiver strain index. *Journal of Gerontology* 38:344–48.

Saleebey D, ed. 1992. *The strengths perspective in social work practice.* New York: Longman.

Schulz R, L Burgio, R Burns, C Eisdorfer, D Gallagher-Thompson, LN Gitlin, and DF Mahoney. 2003. Resources for Enhancing Alzheimer's Caregiver Health (REACH): Overview, site-specific outcomes, and future directions. *Gerontologist* 43:514–20.

Schwentor D and P Brown. 1989, May/June. Assessment of families with a traumatic brain injury relative. *Cognitive Rehabilitation,* 8–20.

Shanas E. 1962. *The health of older people: A social survey.* Cambridge: Harvard University Press.

Shanas E and G Streib, eds. 1965. *Social structure and the family: Generational relations.* Englewood Cliffs, NJ: Prentice-Hall.

Social Policy Research Unit. 2000, November. *Implementing an outcomes approach to carer assessment and review.* York, Eng.: University of York.

Statewide Resources Consultant. 1997, November. *Family caregiver assessment tool: Instruction manual.* San Francisco: Family Caregiver Alliance.

Stone RI. 2000. *Long-term care for the elderly with disabilities: Current policy, emerging trends, and implications for the twenty-first century.* New York: Milbank Memorial Fund.

Switzer GE, SR Wishniewski, SH Belle, R Burns, L Winter, L Thompson, and R Schulz. 2000. Measurement issues in intervention research. In *Handbook on dementia caregiving,* ed. R Schulz, 187–224. New York: Springer.

Teri L, P Truax, R Logsdon, J Uomoto, S Zarit, and PP Vitaliano. 1992. Assessment of behavioral problems in dementia: The revised memory and behavior problems checklist. *Psychology and Aging* 7:622–31.

Tice CJ and K Perkins. 1996. *Mental health issues and aging: Building on the strengths of older persons.* Pacific Grove, CA: Brooks/Cole.

U.S. Department of Health and Human Services. 2002, February 7. HHS awards $128 million in grants to help family caregivers. *HHS News.*

Vitaliano PP, HM Young, and J Russo. 1991. Burden: A review of measures used among caregivers of individuals with dementia. *Gerontologist* 31:67–75.

Weick A, C Rapp, WP Sullivan, and W Kisthardt. 1989. A strengths perspective for social work practice. *Social Work* 34:350–54.

Zarit SH. 1990. Interventions with frail elders and their families: Are they effective and why? In *Stress and coping in later life families*, ed. MAP Stephens, JH Crowther, SE Hobfoll, and DL Tennenbaum, 241–65. New York: Hemisphere.

Zarit SH, NK Orr, and JM Zarit. 1985. *The hidden victims of Alzheimer's disease: Families under stress.* New York: New York University Press.

Zarit SH, KE Reever, and J Bach-Peterson. 1980. Relatives of the impaired elderly: Correlates of feelings of burden. *Gerontologist* 20:649–55.

4

Beyond ADL-IADL: Recognizing the Full Scope of Family Caregiving

Steven M. Albert

SUMMARY

ADL (activities of daily living) and IADL (instrumental activities of daily living) measures fail to capture the work of caregiving in two important respects: they are both too gross and too narrow. These measures are too gross in that they do not specify fully what it means to help with ADLs and IADLs; they are too narrow in that they do not cover the full range of tasks caregivers typically do. For these reasons, ADLs and IADLs will always be an imperfect guide for understanding the realities of caregiving and the needs for assistance.

This chapter proposes a new formulation that builds on four features of the context in which caregiving takes place.

- Timing—whether care is required rarely, frequently but in predictable ways, or frequently in unpredictable, unexpected ways. An example is the central role of nighttime care
- Caregiver proximity—whether it is enough that the caregiver is in the house while someone eats a meal or bathes or must the caregiver be in the same room standing by or providing hands-on help
- Effort—the level of effort required, from coaxing to complete guidance and control

• Participation of the care receiver—whether it is active, passive, or resistant

In the proposed scheme, these features are arrayed against a new organizational grouping of caregiver tasks—skilled nursing care, cognitive support, in-home management, and out-of-home care management. In a fully worked-out system, family caregiver situations could be scored in a way that more fully captures the reality of what caregiving entails.

DESPITE THE UNIVERSAL use of ADL and IADL measures in geriatric assessment (Rodgers and Miller 1997), recent research suggests that these relatively simple measures of older adult competencies do not adequately convey the work carried out by family caregivers (Chapters 1 and 2; Levine et al. 2000). While the measures summarize the care demands of people with health impairments in useful ways, they are less effective in specifying what caregivers do to meet these care demands.

In fairness, we should note that ADL-IADL indicators were never intended to summarize caregiving demands for families. However, policymakers and practitioners have found it convenient to use the measures in this way. They assume that supplying ADL-IADL care is a straightforward response to the care demands or needs cataloged by ADL-IADL status. If ADLs and IADLs summarize the work of caregiving well, as this view suggests, then difficulty in caregiving should be highly related to ADL-IADL status. But a careful look at what caregivers do suggests that the measures fail to capture the work of caregiving in two important respects. ADL-IADL measures are both too gross and too narrow as indicators of caregiving need: too gross in that they do not specify fully what it means to help with ADLs and IADLs and too narrow in that they do not cover the full range of tasks caregivers typically do. For these reasons, ADLs and IADLs will always be an imperfect guide for predicting how hard caregiving is or when families will find it unreasonable or impossible to continue providing such care.

This is an extremely important point, which I develop at length in this chapter. While the ADL-IADL measure tells us that someone has a particular care need, satisfying that need takes place in a wider, more complex environment. Take, for example, bathing. The ADL measure tells us that someone is dependent in bathing. It does not tell us why the person cannot bathe independently, which may involve impairments in mobility and balance or limb weakness or cognitive incapacity or psychiatric disorder. As a result, the ADL measure does not tell us whether the person is cooperative during bathing, whether the person helps wash parts of his or her body once in the tub, or whether the person needs supervision throughout the entire course of bathing or only when getting in and out of the tub. Yet these are the features that make caregiving for someone with a bathing deficit more or less difficult for families.

Thus, while a count of ADL-IADL needs will certainly be correlated with indicators of caregiving challenge (how many hours daily, reported burden and fatigue, risk of nursing home placement), these correlations will be low. Indeed, ADL status explains only a modest amount of the variance in caregiver reports of burden (Chapter 2; Poulshock and Diemling 1984).

The ADL-IADL measures also fail to capture the full context in which families provide care. What kinds of home modifications have family members made to facilitate caregiving? To return to our bathing example, providing bathing care will be easier if families have installed grab bars or have a home with a walk-in shower or flexible shower head. Similarly, what kinds of care arrangements have families put in place to ensure such care if they work or wish to travel or are themselves weak or ill? These too will determine how challenging ADL-IADL care may be. These sorts of care management task are a critical part of the work of caregiving but are not considered in traditional ADL-IADL measures.

Thus, providing care is not simply the mirror image of the need for care expressed in ADL-IADL status. While it is true that caregivers bathe people who need help with bathing, the task of bathing should be considered according to many other dimensions not captured in this ADL measure if we are to understand what caregivers do and hence what makes caregiving challenging.

Rethinking caregiving also requires that we reconsider the distinction between ADL and IADL tasks. The two sets of measures form a rough hierarchy, so that impairment in the more basic ADLs is almost always associated with impairment in the more complex IADLs (Spector et al. 1987). Thus, it is tempting to imagine a single gradient of task complexity and need linking the two domains. But caregiving support for ADL and IADL needs does not seem to share a single, underlying dimension of challenge or difficulty. In fact, the two domains draw on completely different caregiving skills. Help with ADLs, for example, requires physical strength, psychological skill, and perhaps an ability to separate the person from his or her deficit. Help with IADLs requires organizational skill for record keeping, initiative for gathering information related to medical care and benefits, supervisory skill for ensuring that paid helpers maintain a home properly, or even nursing skill, as in medication management.

The great difference in skills required to provide the two types of care suggests that ADLs and IADLs should not be lumped into a single category of caregiving demand. We will see that it is more useful to think of help with ADLs as part of the direct provision of care and help with IADLs as part of other components of caregiving, such as care management (that is, creating and managing a home environment that enables effective caregiving), skilled nursing care (as in medication management), and cognitive support (as in help with using the telephone).

In this chapter, I argue that current ADLs and IADLs are inadequate indicators of care demands and care provision. Building on this discussion, I propose an alternative formulation of family caregiving, which I feel better captures the work of caregiving and may serve as a more adequate job description for family caregiving. I conclude by comparing this expanded definition of family caregiving to the current ADL-IADL–driven approach. I show that ADL-IADL care should be subsumed within a wider, multidomain formulation that gives adequate scope to how people need ADL care and how caregivers develop environments for providing it.

ADL: Inadequate Indicator of Care Demands

To repeat, current ADL measures do not take note of key differences in the way this care is supplied. This limitation is already evident in standard scoring systems. ADLs and IADLs are typically scored with a dichotomous (deficit or no deficit) or three-level ("no, some, or a lot of difficulty" or "no help, some help, or complete help required") indicator, consistent with the presumption that a single gradient of need underlies ADL-IADL competencies. A review of the literature, however, reveals at least four key contextual features that govern how families deliver ADL care. One is timing: whether care is required rarely, frequently but in predictable ways, or frequently in unpredictable, unexpected ways (Montgomery, Gonyea, and Hooyman 1985). A glaring example of the central role of timing is nighttime care; people who routinely need to be taken to the toilet at night, disrupting a caregiver's sleep, are clearly more challenging than people who can be taken to the toilet during the day and sleep through the night, though both equally "need assistance in toileting" (McCluskey 2000). More generally, caregivers forced to adopt care receivers' schedules are likely to be most burdened, as they are most captive to caregiving.

A second dimension is caregiver proximity in the ADL task. Is it enough that a caregiver is in the house while someone eats a meal or bathes or does the caregiver need to be in the same room standing by or does the caregiver have to provide hands-on help? Stand-by help can be quite burdensome in that it limits caregivers to the home even if they do not have to provide hands-on help at all times. In fact, stand-by help in some cases may be more burdensome, since family members need to be available (and hence are prevented from doing other tasks) without a sense that they are providing care. The concept of "vigilance," as described in the Caregiver Vigilance Scale, captures the idea that caregivers see themselves as responsible for the care recipient even when they are not actively providing care (Mahoney et al. 2003).

A third dimension is the kind of effort caregivers need to exert to see that the ADL need is met. Someone with a need for help in bathing may require only supervision or coaxing and support or complete guidance and direction. It is possible that coaxing and support in some cases may be more challenging than complete guidance and control. For example, taking someone to the toilet every two hours may be more burdensome than complete continence care involving disposable diapers.

Finally, it clearly matters whether care receivers participate, actively resist, or passively receive ADL care (Feinstein, Josephy, and Wells 1986); "helping a person who is cooperative is far different from helping a person who is resisting assistance in bathing or eating" (Chapter 2, 43).

These four dimensions give the necessary context to ADL care. The care demands associated with any particular ADL deficit will vary considerably according to the situations defined by these criteria. The dimensions, with representative anchor points, are shown in Table 4.1. These specify the first axis in the expanded definition of caregiving proposed here. Bolded entries indicate the one combination more or less presumed in current ADL-driven approaches to caregiving.

The table shows that any ADL task can be done many ways: in fact, 81 ways, using these 4 dimensions and the 3 levels within each dimension (or 3^4), as shown here. Actually, the number is smaller, since some combinations are likely to be null. For example, it is hard to imagine caregivers being remote or in stand-by capacity for care re-

TABLE 4.1
Axis I, ADL Care

	I. *Timing*	Caregiver Proximity	Caregiver Effort	Care Receiver Response
Axis I Assistance with daily tasks (ADL)	1. Rare, occasional **2. Frequent, predictable** 3. Frequent, unpredictable, disruptive	1. Remote 2. Stand-by **3. Hands-on**	1. Supervision 2. Coaxing **3. Guiding, controlling**	1. Cooperative **2. Passive** 3. Obstructive

ceivers who are obstructive or who need complete guidance and control to perform an ADL task. Similarly, hands-on care implies some degree of contact, so that it is incompatible with limited supervisory effort. Eliminating null combinations would reduce the set of ways to provide ADL care to some 75, still an impressive figure, which gives an idea of how much is left out in the simple ADL specification of "no, some, or a lot of difficulty" or "no help, some help, or complete help required."

The bold entries in the table, then, are only one of many ways to deliver ADL care, but current ADL-driven approaches to caregiving assume that all ADL care is delivered in this way. Policymakers and practitioners assume that ADL care is delivered on a regular schedule and in predictable ways, that caregivers are involved exclusively in a hands-on way, that caregivers take full directive control of the task, and that care receivers are relatively passive in the process. While not stated explicitly, these assumptions undergird the canonical ADL formulation to the extent that ADL measures assume that care needs are habitual and constant, that ADL deficit always implies a need for hands-on help, and that an elder's cognitive or psychiatric status is not relevant for specifying ADL competencies. The table shows, however, that this is a special case of a much more general range of behaviors. In this way, current ADL-driven approaches to caregiving do not do justice to the full range of the ways people need ADL support and hence the full range of ways caregivers provide this care.

ADL: Inadequate Indicator of the Range of Care Provision

Complex Nursing Skills

Direct hands-on care is not limited to help with ADLs. Help to people with chronic disease involves two other major domains of direct care. In addition to axis I, ADL care, I propose "complex nursing care" (axis II) and "cognitive support" (axis III) to cover other major challenges to direct care provision. They are equal in importance to ADL care in every way: in their centrality to a care receiver's health and well-being, in the investment caregivers must make to become skilled as caregivers, and in their difficulty. Yet they are completely neglected in approaches that limit caregiving to provision of ADL support.

Table 4.2 presents the complex nursing care domain, with examples. Caregiver work in this area can again be categorized according to the same dimensions of timing, caregiver proximity, caregiver effort, and care receiver response. However, complex nursing care implies some degree of regularity or fixity in delivery of care and hands-on involvement, restricting the range of values on some of the dimensions. I include in this domain wound care, gastrostomy (feeding tube) and diet care, respiratory care, medication management, monitoring of patient health status, and use of other medical equipment.

Complex nursing care is well described by Reinhard (Chapter 2), who points out that family caregivers are now expected to manage dressing changes, suctioning equipment, oxygen, feeding tubes, catheters, injections, and intravenous therapy—"things that make nursing students tremble." Because complex nursing care implies some degree of fixity in schedule and caregiver involvement, variation in this domain—how hard or easy it is for someone who has already

TABLE 4.2
Axis II, Complex Nursing Care

	II. Timing	**Caregiver Proximity**	**Caregiver Effort**	**Care Receiver Response**
Axis II Complex nursing care				1. Cooperative
Wound care	2. Frequent,			2. Passive
Gastrostomy care/diet	predictable	3. Hands-on	3. Guiding, controlling	3. Obstructive
Respiratory care				
Medications				
Medical monitoring				
Medical equipment				

learned these skills—may largely depend on the care receiver, whether the person is cooperative, passive, or obstructive.

Part of complex nursing skill is monitoring health and knowing when to seek medical intervention or a change in medication regimens. Caregivers report that they become progressively more attuned to recognition of new symptoms and changes in health (Albert 1999). They may become self-perceived health experts, as in the case of the caregiver who claimed she had only one patient, unlike the care receiver's doctor, who had many: "I know when she's sick. I can tell when something's different. You watch bowel movements; diet; nose bleeds; cuts and scratches; sores and bruises. I watch for any kind of cough, cold, and sneeze. You look for different signs" (Albert 1999, 333). One ethnographic study shows that some caregivers reject physician recommendations on the grounds that they feel they understand patient needs better than the physician (Hasselkus 1988). In fact, little is known about the ways family caregivers develop nursing skills. I am also not aware of any studies that have investigated how family caregivers master medical technologies and learn to operate equipment that once was confined to hospital rooms. The little information that is available suggests that much of this learning is informal; caregivers learn from home health nurses, when they take the time to teach them, or are left to gather information on their own (Albert 1999).

Recent survey findings show that formal nursing skills are an important component of family caregiving and that many caregivers are not well prepared to take on the challenge of caregiving. A United Hospital Fund survey (Levine et al. 2000) found that over a third of New York City caregivers did not have formal instruction in using medical equipment and a quarter had no formal instruction in administering medications. A quarter of caregivers in this survey reported they were less than fully capable in helping with prescription medications, changing dressings or bandages, and using medical equipment.

Research also suggests that family caregivers often face the same dilemmas as medical providers, but without the training and professional distance that comes with formal training. In the setting of pain management, Ferrell (2001) reports that family caregivers "made difficult decisions on a daily basis regarding which medicines to give, how much, and when to give analgesics. Family members struggled with titration, when to increase the dose, how to balance relief with side effects, fear of overdosing, and fear of addiction. Family caregivers felt responsible for unrelieved pain." We unfairly expect family caregivers, who usually lack any kind of formal medical or nursing training, to make difficult medical decisions and also to bear responsibility for the consequences of these decisions.

Here too it may be worth making additional distinctions and to ask what is more challenging in this domain: catheter or gastrostomy care, medication titration, or general medical monitoring of patient health? Information is limited, but one might imagine that catheter or feeding-tube care lends itself well to routine, which, once learned, is likely to be easy to maintain. Medication titration and medical monitoring, by contrast, require ongoing judgment and may be more difficult for this reason. It is still unclear how families learn the critical skill of knowing what to ignore and what to watch out for, though the experience of home care paraprofessionals and certified nursing assistants offers some insight in this area (Albert 2001).

Cognitive Support

Cognitive support includes remote and direct supervision, measures to ensure safety, help with cognitive-loaded tasks (such as using the telephone), ongoing efforts to orient care receivers, and attempts to vary the environment to provide stimulation and engagement. Cognitive support also includes management of delirium, agitation, and the psychiatric sequelae of cognitive disorders. Finally, accompanying care receivers with cognitive disorders through medical encounters might also fall within this domain. These forms of support often shade into emotional reassurance, though the latter can be separated from tasks that essentially provide safe and rewarding environments for care receivers with impaired cognition.

Cognitive support is an extremely important component of family care, which is completely ignored in ADL-driven approaches to caregiving. Tasks in this domain lend themselves to the same fourfold characterization according to timing, proximity, effort, and care receiver response, with minor changes, as shown in Table 4.3. Given the nature of cognitive deficit, which is usually not transient (except in the case of delirium), we assume that timing will be predictable and caregiver involvement mostly regular and direct.

Caring for agitated patients may be the most demanding kind of caregiving. In the presence of these extremely difficult behaviors, carrying out personal care tasks, such as bathing and toileting, is far more complicated. Agitated care receivers may hit family caregivers and abuse them verbally. It is also disturbing to see parents or spouses do strange things, such as pull on their skin and injure themselves or tear off their clothing or insist that an ordinary object is something else.

TABLE 4.3
Axis III, Cognitive Support

	III. Timing	Caregiver Proximity	Caregiver Effort	Care Receiver Response
Axis III Cognitive support Supervision Ensuring safety Orientation Stimulation Physician visits Agitation/ behavior management	1. Rare, occa- sional 2. Frequent, predictable	2. Stand-by 3. Hands-on	2. Coaxing 3. Guiding, controlling	1. Cooperative 2. Passive 3. Obstructive

Even when care receivers are not aggressive, just being near someone who is delusional or confused is frightening and can make family members feel strange and uncomfortable.

Family members are well aware of the particular challenges of care for someone with cognitive disorders. Even apart from agitation or obvious psychiatric disorder, these patients may be particularly demanding, as even very simple tasks become difficult and frightening to them. The confusion and disorientation typical of Alzheimer's and other cognitive disorders force caregivers to provide constant supervision but also constant supportive contact. One component of such supportive care is engaging care receivers in activity, when possible, and using the home environment as a source of comfort and guided stimulation. The latter may entail strict routines to "keep things the same every day, over and over; don't change a thing," as one caregiver put it. This kind of crafting of an environment to support family care is a major element in caregiving, however, and deserves separate treatment (see below).

The combination of poor sleep, agitation, and need for constant supervision makes Alzheimer's care extremely difficult. Family caregivers again face the difficult challenge of having to provide nursing and personal assistance care without the professional distance available to nurses and home care paraprofessionals. Successful caregivers, experience shows, are ones who come to adopt advice given by these professionals: "concentrate on the job, not the person" (Albert 2001).

This sort of cognitive support is often hard to separate from efforts to promote emotional health. As one caregiver (quoted in Albert 1999, 333) reported, "You attend to her needs. She needs to feel independent. To make her feel good about herself, you make her look good. Then it's her body: it's got to be clean. And her mind: she's got to be active, visiting people." In this very revealing formulation, "attending to needs" means more than ADL care; it is care for personhood, maintenance of the integrity of the person as a person. We should not lose sight of this insight. Family caregivers provide ADL care not just because a person has ADL deficits but because they wish to maintain a person at his or her highest level of function. This overriding interest leads caregivers to provide a broad environment to support ADL care. I return to this point below.

Finally, I include in cognitive support joint decision-making for the health of care receivers. The most concrete illustration of such joint decision-making (and the best researched element of such care) is active contact with a care receiver's physician. Haug (1994, 2), reviewing the geriatric literature, points out that "we still know very little about doctor-patient-caregiver relationships in terms of the characteristics of the players, content, processes such as initiations, terminations, conflicts, or accommodations, and outcomes." But a number of recent studies now suggest that between 15 and 35 percent of all medical visits of older people involve a family caregiver. In the case of diabetic care for older adults, for example, Silliman (1989; Silliman et al. 1996) found that 36 percent of family members regularly participated in patients' medical encounters. Family members were more likely to participate in medical encounters when patients were older and more frail, and when family members helped patients with daily activities. In a study of 138 family physicians, who saw 4,454 outpatients over two days, Medalie and colleagues (1998) noted that patients were accompanied by family members in 32 percent of visits. Clearly, family caregiver involvement in this component of care will increase in the case of care receivers with greater impairment.

ADL: Inadequate Indicator of Environment in Which Families Provide Care

Providing ADL care requires a special supportive environment. Creating this environment is also part of the work of caregiving. It is impossible to provide help with ADLs if family members cannot lift a care receiver or if they cannot be in the home throughout the day and need to hire someone to fill in for these hours or if the home lacks an essential piece of assistive equipment (such as a sliding board or Hoyer lift) essential for moving the person. Caregivers put these arrangements in place as part of their efforts to provide ADL care. These "care management" activities are no less burdensome or difficult than hands-on ADL care but are not normally considered "ADL." Yet providing such care is impossible without this broader care management activity.

A convenient approach to care management is to distinguish "in-home" and "out-of-home" activities. Within the in-home care management domain fall such tasks as home modification; hiring and supervision of paid home care workers; and purchase, maintenance, and instruction in the use of assistive devices required for ADL care. Within the out-of-home domain fall such tasks as arranging medical care, processing insurance claims, arranging transportation, and putting financial statements together to qualify for entitlements and benefits related to medical disability. The two areas of care management are summarized in Table 4.4. These domains make up axes IV and V of the expanded definition of family caregiving.

The difficulty of care management—the many hours, frustrations, false starts, and steep learning curve experienced by caregivers—has

TABLE 4.4
Axes IV and V, Care Management

	IV. Timing	**Daily Intrusiveness**	*V. Cost* **(Monetary and Opportunity)**
Axis IV			
Care management: in home			
Home modification	1. Intermittent	1. Minimal	1. Minor
Supervision of formal home care, including back-up	2. Ongoing	2. Considerable	2. Major
		3. Intolerable	
Other equipment			
Axis V			
Care management: out of home			
Arranging medical care, appointments	1. Intermittent	1. Minimal	1. Minor
	2. Ongoing	2. Considerable	2. Major
Insurance claims		3. Intolerable	
Transportation			
Financial planning			

been described anecdotally (Brody 2004; Levine 2000) but never subjected, as far as I know, to systematic analysis. For the in-home component, perhaps the most well-described challenge is the difficulty of hiring and supervising paid home care providers. Many caregivers have never had supervisory experience; they may be ill-equipped to interview potential employees and define job responsibilities. Or they may find that they spend so much time teaching home care providers how to do their jobs that they would be better off without such help.

Paid home care support is a mixed blessing in other ways as well. Having a stranger in the home is intrusive. Paid home care providers face the difficult job of doing "family work" without being family, a recipe for misunderstanding and conflict (Albert 2001; Levine 2000). Families find it difficult to draw distinctions between a home care provider's "care time" and their own family time. We can add to these challenges the inherent difficulty of finding someone able to meet family standards of sensitivity and respect for a person's preferences. If family members provide ADL care to maintain the person-hood of a family member, they expect paid home care providers to do the same, adding additional tension to an already difficult relationship. The issues are further complicated by the unreliability of some home care agencies and employees; their inadequate training, low pay, and high turnover; and all the other ills of an industry that has still not managed to assume the critical role in long-term care required of it.

As mentioned earlier, in the proposed expanded definition of family caregiving, many tasks normally considered IADLs fall within the care management domain. For example, impaired people receiving ADL support (especially older adults with cognitive disorders) may have difficulty using the telephone to arrange transportation or schedule a medical appointment. They may have difficulty completing an insurance claim, clarifying the hours and schedules of formal caregivers provided by a home care agency, and arranging for delivery of medical equipment and assistive devices. These tasks—using the telephone, managing personal finances, arranging transportation, and accompanying a care receiver so he or she can get to places outside of walking distance—are part of care management and hence inherent in the provision of ADL care. The same would be true for laundry and meal preparation insofar as a care receiver's medical status requires a particular environment for ADL care, such as a special diet or frequent washing of clothes and bed linens. The category of care management thus includes much of the supportive work caregivers provide for IADLs.

I propose three dimensions to specify the challenge of care management tasks (see Table 4.4). These tasks will be more or less difficult according to timing, intrusiveness, and cost. Tasks may be intermittent or ongoing, be variably intrusive, and require major or minor investments in time or monetary resources. Together, these dimensions offer a plausible way to categorize care management according to likely burden.

Comparison of Standard and Expanded Definitions of Family Caregiving

To repeat, the ADL-driven definition of family caregiving is limited to axis I of the proposed expanded definition. Moreover, typical approaches to ADLs do not consider the behavioral complexity of providing help with these tasks: they do not distinguish between stand-by and active hands-on help, for example, or between care that is easy to provide because care receivers cooperate and care that is nearly impossible to provide because care receivers are agitated and resistive.

It is hard to imagine caregiving situations, however, in which caregivers provide only axis I, ADL support. People in need of bathing support or help with toileting will certainly require some care management support (axes IV and V), even if they do not require complex nursing care (axis II) or cognitive support (axis III). In fact, little empirical information is available on this point: how often is ADL care associated with a need for complex nursing care, cognitive support, or care management activity? Available data suggest great overlap between ADL deficit and cognitive impairment among older adults, but the association is less clear for younger, impaired populations.

With a team of researchers, I investigated this overlap in a sample of family caregivers to people with traumatic brain injury (see Albert et al. 2002 for a complete description of this sample). Returning to these data, we defined each of the five axes using an appropriate indicator. Axis I, ADL care, was defined in terms of need for help in dressing. Axis II, skilled nursing care, was defined by caregiver administration of medications. Axis III, cognitive support, was defined by caregiver reports regarding the frequency with which the person with brain injury was confused. Axis IV, in-home care management, was defined in terms of caregiver reports of satisfaction with paid personal assistance providers. Axis V, out-of-home care management, was defined by reports of difficulty filing insurance claims related to medical care for the care receiver. For these analyses we used all interview occasions in which caregivers reported information for the different indicators.

In this sample of caregivers to people with brain injury, 47 percent were providing ADL support and 71 percent medication management support; 41 percent reported that care receivers were confused at times. Thirty-five percent of those with formal, paid help reported dissatisfaction with this help, and 36 percent reported need for help completing insurance claims. About 20 percent of the caregivers did not report current help in any of the domains, largely because care receivers were still in the brain injury unit or in nursing homes awaiting discharge.

Table 4.5 shows the correlation matrix for the five indicators. Note that the sample for the paid formal care ($n = 67$) indicator is less than the sample for other indicators ($n = 150$–160). Included in the table is one measure of caregiver burden or likely burnout, the extent to which caregivers in this sample reported they were "overwhelmed" and not sure they could continue as caregivers.

In this sample, caregiving for many families clearly involves all five types of work included in the expanded definition. The pattern of correlations suggests that family members performing one kind of caregiving work are likely to be involved in the others as well, though to varying degrees. The strongest association is between axes I and II, ADL tasks and complex nursing care ($r = .70$), as referenced by providing help with dressing and providing help with medication dispensing. This finding is consistent with the hierarchical relationship between IADL and ADL tasks, in which ADL deficit almost always implies IADL deficit (Chapter 2). Axis III tasks, or need for cognitive support (as indexed by reports of patient confusion), are associated with both ADL ($r = .40$) and complex nursing tasks ($r = .48$). In-home (as referenced by satisfaction with paid personal assistance help) and out-of-home (as referenced by need for help preparing insurance claims) care management have variable associations with each of the three direct-care domains. The two care management do-

TABLE 4.5

Correlations across Five Caregiver Axes and with Caregiver Burden

	1	2	3	4	5	6
1. Help with dressing Axis I	1.0					
2. Medication supervision Axis II	.70**	1.0				
3. Patient confusion Axis III	.40**	.48**	1.0			
4. Satisfaction with in- home paid caregivers Axis IV (subset)	.08	.24*	.21*	1.0		
5. Insurance claims Axis V	.22**	.28**	.37**	.26**	1.0	
6. Caregiver overwhelmed	.33**	.28**	.18	.36**	.29**	1.0

*p < .01
**p < .001

mains are modestly but significantly correlated with cognitive support ($r = .24, .28$) and complex nursing care ($r = .21, .37$). Out-of-
home care management was associated with ADL care ($r = .22$). In-
home care management was less clearly connected to ADL care, but
this last correlation should be considered in the light of its restriction
to families with formal, paid home care and therefore to a sample of
care receivers with little variation in ADL deficit.

This analysis suggests that the five axes of caregiving work are related; caregivers providing support in one domain are likely to be providing support, to a variable degree, in the other domains as well.
While family caregiving does not entail work in all five areas for all
cases, it is notable, as the last row of Table 4.5 shows, that all five areas are associated with caregiver reports of burden. These bivariate
correlations extend over a considerable range (.18–.36). Notably, ADL
support and in-home care management were most highly related to
reports from caregivers that they are overwhelmed and unable to continue much longer in their role. Indeed, in multiple regression analy-

ses for this sample, these two domains are independent, significant predictors of such burden. Using all five types of caregiving work as predictors of burden for the subset of caregivers with paid help, we find significant independent associations for ADL and both types of care management work. Since standard approaches to caregiving consider only ADL and not care management, it is not surprising that ADL severity is no more than a modest predictor of caregiver burden.

Conclusion: How an Expanded Definition of Family Caregiving May Help Identify Limits to Family Caregiving

The expanded definition of family caregiving proposed here shows that ADL care is only one element of what falls within the rubric of "family caregiving." I suggest that ADL care should be subsumed within a wider, multidomain formulation that gives adequate scope to how people need ADL care and how caregivers develop environments for providing it. I propose four additional axes for describing the work of caregiving: skilled nursing care, cognitive support, in-home care management, and out-of-home care management. In a fully worked-out system for describing family caregiving, family situations could be scored on each of five axes, shown in Figure 4.1. The result would be a fuller description that captures the reality of what families do as caregivers.

In this effort, I have been guided by family caregivers themselves, who recognize that ADL support requires not just direct care provision but also development of an environment for the delivery of this care. Providing such an environment is "care management." Care management includes all the auxiliary tasks that allow a home to become a reasonable and effective setting for the provision of ADL support. Data from a sample of caregivers to people with brain injury suggest that these care management tasks may be as burdensome as direct ADL support.

FIGURE 4.1
Expanded Caregiving Domain

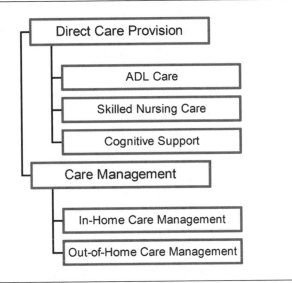

I also note that direct ADL support often comes with allied but distinct caregiving tasks, which I include in the domains of skilled nursing care and cognitive support. In the current ADL-driven approach to caregiving, these domains are hidden sources of unmeasured variance within particular ADLs. But full recognition of what caregivers do requires that we identify these domains, first, because families are now expected to take on skilled nursing care tasks and, second, because families will continue to provide dementia care for an increasingly older population.

The behavioral complexity of ADL support also suggests further qualification of the ADL component of caregiving. "Providing ADL support" is inadequately described unless we know something about the timing of such care, the spatial proximity of caregivers when they provide such care, the effort required, and the response of the people who receive such care. Without specification in these terms, we simply will not understand the true demands of ADL support.

Finally, in developing an expanded definition of family caregiving, I followed the lead of caregivers, who speak of "attending to someone's needs" as requiring far more than ADL care. Family caregivers provide ADL care because they wish to maintain a person at his or her highest level of function, not just because a person needs help with bathing, dressing, or toileting. This overriding interest leads caregivers to try to provide a broad environment to support ADL care that is stimulating or protective and includes social engagement and other elements that fall in the realm of cognitive support.

What would it mean to consider family caregiving using this expanded definition? A first step would be to devise a scoring system that allows classification of family situations along the five proposed axes. I have suggested one such scoring system here. In this way, the true burden of family care could be measured. Second, scoring family care along the five axes will enable us to understand better why families, given the same ADL challenge and same set of resources, differ in their thresholds for exiting from caregiving and their ability to adapt more or less effectively to its challenges. Expanding the definition of caregiving in this way should allow better measurement of the stress of family caregiving. Finally, it may be possible to use the five-axis system proposed here to establish a more fine-grained way to target resources for families. For example, families scoring high in three or more of the domains might be good candidates for respite; alternatively, families scoring high in ADL support only, with little challenge in the other domains, might be less likely to benefit from respite or other interventions.

The expanded definition of family caregiving proposed here, I suggest, is an appropriate way to measure the "demand" side of caregiving: what services caregivers must provide to address the needs of family members who are frail, disabled, or ill. Missing is a comparable measure of "caregiving supply": what resources caregivers need to meet each of these demands. Both sets of measures are required if we are to understand whether any particular family is likely to succeed as a caregiving unit.

The expanded definition proposed here has the advantage of recognizing the true complexity of family care. For this reason it is likely to be useful for understanding the limits of family care: what should be considered reasonable and what unreasonable demands on caregivers.

References

Albert SM. 1999. The caregiver as part of the dementia management team. *Disease Management Health Outcomes* 5:329–37.

———. 2001. Personal assistants speak about home care: A guide to home care, spoken by the women who provide personal assistance/home attendant care to frail elders in New York City. Typescript.

Albert SM, A Im, L Brenner, M Smith, and R Waxman. 2002. Effect of a social work liaison program on family caregivers to people with brain injury. *Journal of Head Trauma Rehabilitation* 17:175–89.

Brody EM. 2004. *Women in the middle: Their parent care years.* 2nd ed. New York: Springer.

Feinstein AR, BR Josephy, and CK Wells. 1986. Scientific and clinical problems in indexes of functional disability. *Annals of Internal Medicine* 105:413–20.

Ferrell B. 2001. Pain observed: The experience of pain from the family caregiver's perspective. *Clinics in Geriatric Medicine* 17:595–609.

Hasselkus BR. 1988. Meaning in family caregiving: Perspectives on caregiver-professional relationships. *Gerontologist* 28:686–91.

Haug M. 1994. Elderly patients, caregivers, and physicians: Theory and research on health care triads. *Journal of Health and Social Behavior* 35:1–12.

Levine C, ed. 2000. *Always on call: When illness turns families into caregivers.* New York: United Hospital Fund.

Levine C, AN Kuerbis, DA Gould, M Navaie-Waliser, PH Feldman, and K Donelan. 2000. *A survey of family caregivers in New York City: Findings and implications for the health care system.* New York: United Hospital Fund.

Mahoney DF, RN Jones, DW Coon, AB Mendelsohn, LN Gitlin, and M Ory. 2003, January/February. The Caregiver Vigilance Scale: Application and validation in the Resources for Enhancing Alzheimer's Caregiver Health (REACH) project. *American Journal of Alzheimer's Disease and Other Dementias* 18(1):39–48.

McCluskey A. 2000. Paid attendant carers hold important and unexpected roles which contribute to the lives of people with brain injury. *Brain Injury* 14:943–57.

Medalie JH, SJ Zyzanski, D Langa, and KC Stange. 1998. The family in family practice: Is it a reality? *Journal of Family Practice* 146:390–96.

Montgomery RJV, JG Gonyea, and NR Hooyman. 1985. Caregiving and the experience of subjective and objective burden. *Family Relations* 34:19–26.

Poulshock SW and GT Diemling. 1984. Families caring for elders in residence: Issues in the measurement of burden. *Journal of Gerontology* 39:230–39.

Rodgers W and B Miller. 1997. A comparative analysis of ADL questions in surveys of older people. *Journal of Gerontology* 52B (special issue):21–36.

Silliman RA. 1989. Caring for the frail older patient: The doctor-patient-caregiver relationship. *Journal of General Internal Medicine* 4:237–41.

Silliman RA, S Bhatti, A Khan, KA Dukes, and LM Sullivan. 1996. The care of older persons with diabetes mellitus: Families and primary care physicians. *Journal of the American Geriatrics Society* 44:1314–21.

Spector WD, S Katz, LB Murphy, and JP Fulton. 1987. The hierarchical relationship between activities of daily living and instrumental activities of daily living. *Journal of Chronic Diseases* 140:481–89.

5

You Can't Get There from Here: Dimensions of Caregiving and Dementias of Policymaking

Bruce C. Vladeck

SUMMARY

The process of fleshing out the dimensions of caregiving and caregivers' needs in the previous chapters highlights how little specificity about their characteristics and needs surfaces in most discussions of long-term care policy. The conceptual and political context in which such analyses would be most useful hardly exists, and even in its current primitive form that context does not command any sort of consensus among policymakers or the general public.

This chapter points out some basic questions that need to be answered:

- Which caregivers should receive help?
- What kind of help should they receive?
- Should support for caregivers be universal or highly targeted or somewhere in between?
- Who should decide which caregivers get help, and what kind?

While we are a long way away from a coherent long-term care policy that would address the needs of caregivers, some actions in the near term would be a partial response:

- Paid providers of formal in-home services should be required to consult regularly with informal caregivers about their own resources and needs, as well as those of the patient.

- Medicare- and Medicaid-paid home care services, for which formal patient assessments are already required, should strengthen and expand the assessment of caregiver capabilities and needs.
- Caregiver assessments should be a mandatory part of the patient assessment process for Medicaid home- and community-based waivers.
- Medicare and JCAHO (Joint Commission for the Accreditation of Healthcare Organizations) standards for hospital discharge planning should be strengthened to require caregiver assessment, using a standard instrument, and the results incorporated into the discharge plan.

FOR MANY YEARS, those concerned with long-term care for the elderly and disabled have been well aware of the central role played by family caregivers. "Informal caregivers," it has long been recognized, are the sole or primary source of care for as many as 80 percent or more of community residents who are unable to fully care for themselves. Yet until recently, the primary public policy question that the importance of family caregivers seemed to raise was how to design public supports for "formal" care in ways that minimize the associated reduction in informal services, even though several generations of data have suggested that such displacement is relatively rare and of limited magnitude. Or to put the issue more bluntly, policymakers have perceived the problem as one of trying to avoid paying for something they have become accustomed to getting free. Among the politer characterizations of this anxiety has been the so-called woodwork effect: the belief that expansion in the availability of in-home services would bring "out of the woodwork" many potential clients previously unknown to the formal systems.

More recently, thanks in large part to some remarkably effective advocacy on the part of a relatively small number of caregivers and their advocates, many policymakers have come to accept the idea that some form of assistance to caregivers would be not only simply fair but also financially prudent as a way of preventing much higher expenditures that might be necessitated if the caregivers became incapacitated or unavailable. Proposals to provide various forms of support to family caregivers have proliferated, and some have even evolved into modest initial programs.

As the issue of formal supports for caregivers has received increasingly sympathetic attention, a whole host of issues has arisen about how policies providing such supports should be defined, designed, and administered. The first four chapters in this volume focus on one of the central design issues: how to appropriately and efficiently describe what caregivers actually do in the performance of their roles, as a starting point to determine what kinds of help they might need, on an instrumental, daily level and in the long term to allow them to maintain their caregiving roles. A more accurate and up-to-date description than the conventional activities of daily living (ADLs) and instrumental activities of daily living (IADL) measures, these authors argue, is important as a basis for identifying what services or benefits caregivers should receive. But at least for this reader, the very sophistication and level of detail in these chapters, in the context of current discussions of long-term care and support for caregivers, seem somehow sadly incongruous. The very process of fleshing out the dimensions of caregiving and caregivers' needs highlights how little specificity about the characteristics and needs of the clients in need of care governs most discussions of long-term care policy. The sad fact is that the conceptual and political context in which such analyses would be most useful hardly exists, and even in current primitive form that context comes nowhere near to commanding any sort of consensual acceptance among policymakers or the general public.

It is a truism to say that we have no coherent policy for long-term care in this country, but we do not, even though annual public spending on long-term care is measured in figures with 11 or 12 digits—and if we take the literature on caregiving seriously, those numbers are dwarfed by the almost totally uncompensated costs borne by family caregivers. We have no consensus on who should receive services and how those services should be paid for, or on what the role of government should be in allocating and paying for services. There is almost universal consensus that people in need of long-term care services should be able to receive them at home, but little understanding of just what that means, or whether in fact it always makes sense.

Thinking about caregiving is even more ill-formed and inchoate. There appears to be a consensus that informal caregiving is a good thing, that what caregivers do merits approbation and possibly formal support, that caregiving can be quite stressful on a number of dimensions and that caregivers themselves could often benefit from various forms of assistance, and that it might be fiscally rational or morally desirable (or possibly even both) to develop public programs to provide caregivers with some of the support they need. But it is a long way from that consensus to policy design. Some very elemental questions still need to be answered.

- Which caregivers should receive help?
- What kind of help should they receive?
- Should support for caregivers be universal or highly targeted or somewhere in between?
- Who should decide which caregivers get help, and what kind?

All of these questions, I submit, need to be addressed if the lessons contained in the four preceding chapters are to be put to productive use in the policy process.

Who Should Be Helped?

Except for the growing number of people who live alone (a category that includes those with the greatest need for long-term care services, but about whom there is substantially less conceptual confusion), most adults and a surprisingly large number of adolescent and preadolescent children engage regularly in activities—from shopping and meal preparation to housecleaning to management of medical care and provision of simple health services—on behalf of the people with whom they live (and themselves) that would qualify as "caregiving" if one or more of the beneficiaries of those services were to be classified as a care recipient in some formal scheme or other. The critical point is this: the boundary between ordinary family or quasi-family life and "caregiving" of the sort discussed in these chapters requires some classification or labeling of the care recipient as well. To take a purely hypothetical example, if I bring my wife breakfast in bed, I may be displaying significant conjugal considerateness (and prudence), but I become a caregiver only if she has assumed a role of sickness or dependence.

The dependency role of the care recipient is thus part of the definition of what makes one a caregiver. That is why caregiving for one's children can became so fraught with tension as they gradually seek to free themselves from (at least explicit) dependency and assert their own autonomy and independence. And to stay with the issue of caregiving for children for one moment longer, it is also noteworthy, and relevant, that the United States has long been distinguished among the industrialized nations of the West for the paucity of its public subsidies for those taking care of children, especially young children. This historical tightfistedness in subsidies for child care is yet another part of the context in which the new discussions of caregivers for the elderly and disabled is taking place.

Even though some formal attribution of dependency (for which ADLs, for all their well-documented inadequacies, remain the standard metric) is a precondition for the receipt of insurance benefits or public assistance for the elderly and disabled, many of those beneficiaries are themselves eager to minimize their dependency, in apparent if not real terms. This desire often creates tension between caregiver and care recipient, but more to the point, it creates a certain ambiguousness in the caregiver's role, since the more successful the caregiver is at assisting the patient to become independent, the more the legitimacy of his or her distinct role as caregiver may be called into question. Only when some dimensions of a client's dependency can be established by incontrovertible physical fact, as in the case of younger, wheelchair-bound physically disabled people, are policymakers and the public sometimes comfortable with the notion that the recipients of care should play a major role in directing services to maximize their independence.

Determination of which caregivers should receive help would be more straightforward if we had more rational systems for determining which potential clients should receive help. ADLs are often discussed as criteria for the receipt of formal services, but even they are only occasionally used for that purpose. The criteria for receipt of Medicare-covered in-home services are notoriously opaque, variable in interpretation, and often irrelevant to commonsense understanding of what people need; and each state, of course, has its own rules to determine eligibility for Medicaid-covered home care, most of which have a considerable subjective component. In general, to be eligible for comprehensive, Medicaid-covered, community-based services, beneficiaries need to be determined to be sufficiently disabled to require nursing home care, but just what that means varies not only from state to state but often from one assessor to the next.

Advocates of expanded public support for caregivers frequently point, with good reason, to the Medicare hospice program as the one federally defined benefit that explicitly provides for services to caregivers, although those are quite limited. And the hospice benefit would seem to have about as clear-cut an eligibility criterion as one would want: terminal illness, with expected survival of six months or less. But even that criterion often turns out to be quite difficult to apply in practice and has been subject to extensive criticism—in addition to a few well-publicized instances of abuse.

If we had universal benefits for long-term care anywhere in the United States, these problems would be less pervasive; or, put more accurately, in the context of universal benefits it would be necessary to develop some more objective and defensible criteria for determining who gets what. But eligibility for publicly supported benefits is likely to remain a shifting amalgam of client medical conditions, client functional capabilities and potential, client and family income, and client and family resources—including the availability of unassisted caregivers. In that circumstance, developing any sort of rational algorithms for identifying the caregivers who merit public support is essentially impossible.

What Kind of Help Should Caregivers Receive?

The growing body of literature on caregiving, including the preceding chapters in this volume, describe two separate—although not mutually incompatible—sorts of assistance that caregivers might receive. Caregivers might be provided assistance to permit them to perform their caregiving more effectively, more efficiently, less stressfully, or for a longer time—if respite or other services prevent burnout and total exhaustion. Or caregivers might be compensated for their caregiving, either directly through payment of one sort or another or indirectly through the provision of goods or services—or even, in at least one proposed program, of credits toward future care receipt.

Assistive services in the first category generally presume (without asking) that the caregiver accepts the role into which he or she has been placed and can and will sustain that role if only a little help is judiciously applied. Many caregivers could clearly benefit from better education and information about the condition and needs of the care recipient and the specific services they are assumed or expected to provide, especially when those services involve considerable technological or clinical complexity. Respite care would be a boon for many. But a complete assessment of the assistance needs of many caregivers would undoubtedly identify many instances in which the only sensible form of assistance would be that provided by a paid, nonfamily, "formal" caregiver. And that would, in turn, immediately raise the question of the extent to which responsibility for total care of the care recipient should be allocated between the formal and informal mechanisms.

Caregivers with considerable financial resources make such allocation decisions by themselves all the time, of course, but few caregivers have that level of resources, so we are immediately back to the very difficult and—in most of this country—largely unresolved issue of the extent and nature of public responsibility for the care of frail and disabled persons in the community. And recognition of the legitimate needs of caregivers only complicates efforts to achieve policy consensus on the overall size of the public role, since in any given case the least-cost strategy would be to provide the absolute minimum level of formal services necessary to encourage or induce the informal caregiver to remain as involved as possible, while considerations of equity and simple fairness might suggest making more formal services available in response to greater efforts by informal caregivers.

Caregivers' advocates have made a number of efforts to estimate the magnitude of the economic contribution of caregivers, and while one may cavil with the specific estimating methods, there is no question that many caregivers incur considerable financial sacrifice by forgoing or altering employment or by limiting their participation in other potentially economically beneficial activities, such as education or training. Proposals to provide some form of remuneration to caregivers—either directly or, more commonly, by resort to that currently preferred cure-all to all public policy problems, tax credits—have, perhaps predictably, proliferated.

One might be tempted to raise the philosophical question whether it is desirable to monetize what has historically been seen and felt, in many circumstances, as a normal extension of ordinary family relationships, in which family members take care of one another in ways that have hardly ever been symmetrical. But in contemporary U.S. policy discourse, everything is subject to monetization, so the more pressing question becomes one of how levels of compensation for caregivers are to be established. Should they be equivalent to what formal caregivers are paid? On one hand, given how little formal caregivers are paid in most communities, making the compensation equivalent would still create a significant financial sacrifice for many informal caregivers who must forgo better-paying employment, while obliterating any presumed program savings obtained from having informal services available to substitute for paid caregivers. On the other hand, in the absence of training and licensure requirements for informal caregivers, and the presumably greater psychic income they receive from taking care of loved ones, it hardly seems fair to pay them more than formal caregivers.

In a society in which most women are now expected to be economically self-sufficient, but in which economic equity for women is still (at best) a distant aspiration, and in which most caregiving is provided by middle-aged and older women, there is no real solution to this dilemma within the confines of the caregiving issue itself. Only a more systematic effort to redress gender inequities in compensation and the distribution of wealth could provide a context for more rational approaches to the question of compensating caregivers. In this regard, it might be suggested that only in the United States could politicians claim to have accomplished something by providing for unpaid family medical leave. But the fact is that caregivers are disproportionately concentrated in low-wage, low-benefit employment for which any absence from work creates an economic hardship. If working women had, on average, the same vacation and personal-leave benefits as working men, the economic consequences of caregiving would be much less severe.

The whole question of compensating caregivers also points to one of the other basic lacunae in discussions of caregiving in the United States—the fact that our major public programs that subsidize long-term care and other in-home caregiving are based in individual entitlements. Thus, when Lynn Friss Feinberg (Chapter 3) describes caregiver needs assessment in other countries, she rightly emphasizes the extent to which the needs of the primary care recipient and the family caregiver or caregivers should logically be assessed together. Caregiving is something that takes place, by and large, within families, and that fact needs to be understood in the context of the resources, attributes, and needs of those households. But as noted above, social welfare policy in the United States tends to focus on atomized individuals, not on families; we support the former but only rarely the latter.

Universal or Targeted Benefits?

On any given day, there are probably between five and six million Americans engaged in relatively demanding caregiving for family members or close friends who are old and frail, or young and disabled. The majority of those care recipients are probably unknown to agencies with formal responsibilities for long-term or continuing care of the elderly or disabled in their communities, although they are undoubtedly in frequent contact with individual providers of medical and health-related services. Accepting for the moment that there should be some mechanism for providing assistance to at least some caregivers, the issue of which caregivers should receive that assistance must be confronted.

One option would be to provide assistance to every caregiver who meets some minimum threshold of eligibility. In the absence of adequate care delivery and needs assessment infrastructure in most U.S. communities, the only way to do that in the near future would probably be through some form of cash assistance. In such a program, the likelihood of a good "fit" between the needs of any particular caregiver and the nature of the assistance would be minimized, and the expense would undoubtedly be quite considerable—mitigated only by whatever administrative barriers to receipt of the benefit emerged, and thus the number of otherwise eligible beneficiaries who would not be helped. At the other extreme, one could minimize public expenditures by limiting caregiver assistance to those instances in which the care recipient was already receiving publicly supported services, with the specific help provided to caregivers set in such a way as to minimize paid caregiving expense. Or, to take what are now the most popular policy proposals, and those with the greatest likelihood of enactment in the near term, one could provide financial subsidies in inverse proportion to the needs of caregiving households, by distributing those subsidies through a system of tax credits (in a world in which roughly half of households headed by someone 65 and older do not currently file federal income tax returns).

Any policy proposal located almost anywhere along this spectrum would require some determination of who should be eligible for benefits, but under existing circumstances, it is hard to imagine that any of them would require assessments of the depth or sophistication discussed in the four preceding chapters. Sophisticated needs assessment methodologies make sense only in conjunction with policies that permit relatively sophisticated responses to particular needs.

Who Should Decide?

The most advanced methods for assessing caregivers' needs, as described in this volume, are administered in conjunction with programs that lodge responsibility for overseeing and allocating long-term care resources for substantial populations in defined geographic communities. In other words, they are all found in other countries. In the United States, we have only one state, Oregon, and a few other communities in which a single agency has responsibility for all publicly financed long-term care services for the elderly, and even in the exceptional case of Oregon other homebound recipients of public benefits are not covered. Nor are services provided through private insurance mechanisms or private family resources integrated into the Oregon system.

It seems, indeed, safe to say that we lack public consensus in most of the United States about just what the role of the public sector should be in overseeing services for the chronically ill and disabled in the community, even when the great preponderance of those services are purchased with public funds. There are a number of models of communitywide public services management for individuals with specific kinds of problems—such as chronic mental illness or developmental disabilities—but fewer models providing care to the far more numerous population of the frail elderly, and none, as far as I know, that incorporates oversight of privately paid services in the same system.

Medicaid, by far the largest source of financing for in-home and community-based services for people with chronic illnesses or disability, is simply not designed, by basic statutory or administrative structure, to manage the formal care, let alone the full spectrum of formal and informal services, of defined populations. Under both demonstration and home- and community-based waiver authorities, states have labored mightily for a generation to develop mechanisms to provide such service allocation and care management, but even today only a small fraction of Medicaid-paid services are delivered through such mechanisms. Medicare lags far behind. A minority of private insurers and health plans do a better job, but the populations they serve are relatively minuscule. And in a still larger context, it seems probable that the combination of fiscal stresses on the states and Republican hegemony in Washington may lead, in the short term at least, to a retrenchment in existing Medicaid services.

In the absence of appropriate service allocation structures, mechanisms for assessing caregiver needs can serve a valuable educational purpose and can help produce invaluable research, but their practical utility is likely to be limited. And experience seems to suggest that caregiving organizations and professionals can be expected to collect sophisticated assessment information only to the extent that their reimbursement or other benefits depend on it. However desirable the collection of such information might be, in other words, requiring such collection might not be the most realistic strategy.

Conclusions: Toward a Short-Term Agenda for Caregiving and Caregiver Needs Assessment

Taking the dimensions of caregiving seriously is only a reminder of how far the current U.S. policy process is from any serious attempt to tackle the problems of the chronically ill and disabled residing in our communities, even as the numbers of people with those needs continue to mushroom. Not only are we not systematically evaluating and enumerating the needs of caregivers; we are not even systematically evaluating and enumerating the needs of the care recipients or potential care recipients themselves, except for the highly skewed subset of those who receive Medicare home care benefits or services from a few Medicaid waiver programs or managed care plans. And even in those instances, provider complaints about "regulatory burden" are likely to reduce, rather than improve, the scope of assessments in the near future. Perhaps focusing on caregiving can help identify and mobilize a political constituency influential enough to impel providers and policymakers to take all of these issues more seriously, although it is hard to find the data to support such optimism.

In the meantime, while efforts to develop or improve systems of care for the chronically ill and disabled seem mired in the long-standing stasis in U.S. health policy, the very tangible needs of literally millions of caregivers are going unmet every day, and it is both insufficient and cavalier to respond to those needs by concluding that nothing can be done. In fact, while we are a long way away (and possibly growing farther from, not closer to, the goal) from implementation of more rational systems of care in many U.S. communities that would include adequate supports for informal caregivers, there are probably some things that can and should be done in the shorter term, to respond in at least a partial way to needs that are already out there. I suggest the following potential agenda:

- Paid providers of formal in-home services, such as home health agencies, should be required to consult regularly with informal caregivers about their own resources and needs, as well as those of the patients. A radical but probably desirable extension of this effort would be a requirement that the primary informal caregiver, when one is present, participate in the formulation of the patient's care plan, since he or she will undoubtedly be expected to participate in all sorts of ways in its implementation.

- In conjunction with the first recommendation, for Medicare- and Medicaid-paid home care services, for which formal patient assessments are already required, assessment of caregiver capabilities and needs should be strengthened and expanded. This suggestion will undoubtedly generate vociferous opposition from the home-care community, which already considers the OASIS (Outcomes and Assessment Information Set) assessment process overly burdensome, and which has campaigned with some success to weaken it.

- Caregiver assessments should be a mandatory part of the patient assessment process for Medicaid home- and community-based waiver programs, and those programs should be encouraged to add services to caregivers to the repertoire of services they offer and manage.

- Medicare and JCAHO standards for discharge planning (which are fairly universally ignored by providers and surveyors) should be strengthened to require caregiver assessment using a standard instrument, and incorporation of the results of that assessment into the discharge plan—and those requirements should then be enforced.

All of these recommendations would be likely to produce consider-able resistance and opposition from the provider community, but if we are serious about recognizing the needs of informal caregivers, they could contribute far more to meeting those needs than any of the largely cosmetic proposals now so popular among politicians of all stripes. If we are going to take caregiving and caregivers seriously, these would be serious—if very limited and incremental—steps.

6

Measuring What Matters: Levers for Change

David A. Gould

SUMMARY

The previous detailed and comprehensive chapters have pointed out that ADLs and IADLs fail to capture not only the complexities of family caregiving but often its very essence. If we can successfully reframe the way caregiving is defined and understood, we can move ahead with the hard work of designing more responsive services, educational programs, and public policies.

Four areas that call for further exploration and experimentation are research, professional education, public and caregiver education, and public policy.

Research is needed to devise and validate more accurate definitions of caregiver activities, create a more holistic framework for the caregiving experience, understand the management aspects of caregiving, grapple with the commonalities and differences experienced by caregivers, come to a consensus on caregiver assessment methods and practices, and deal with quality of care. The information garnered from these sources should be the springboard for developing new and more sensitive programs to train, support, and counsel caregivers.

Even the best designed, most rigorous research studies will not change practice unless health care and social service professionals are aware of the implications for their daily interactions with family caregivers. Education at all levels and for all disciplines should include familiarity with research findings, discussion about aspects of family caregiving, and opportunities to interact with caregivers.

Public education is an essential part of changing the environment in which family caregiving goes on. It can take many forms: television, articles in newspapers and periodicals, community forums, discussions in religious settings, and volunteer activities.

Public policy should be approached with an eye to achieving both short-term and long-term goals. Improving the transition process from hospital to home by strengthening discharge planning and enforcing rules already in place should be a short-term priority.

THE LARGELY INVISIBLE activities of family caregivers constitute one of the most pervasive and enduring sources of support for people who need assistance of various kinds because of frailty, illness, or disability. The formal health care system could not be sustained without the enormous contribution of family caregivers. Thus, a better understanding of the nature of this phenomenon is of vital importance to health care in the United States.

The thesis of this book is straightforward: because so much of what family caregivers do takes place outside health care institutions or physicians' offices, away from the experience of health care and social service professionals, it is deemed "informal," unpaid work. As a result, too little attention has been given to consistently or accurately measuring what constitutes this informal care. By default, activities of daily living (ADLs) and instrumental activities of daily living (IADLs) have become universal descriptors of family caregiving; yet, as the authors in the preceding detailed and comprehensive chapters point out, these measures fail to capture not only the complexities of caregiving but often its very essence.

Since caregiving is essentially a labor of love, duty, or necessity, why is it important to reframe the way we categorize and measure it? Doesn't such an effort detract from the intimate nature of family relationships? On the contrary, such a reframing can help us understand, value, and better support family caregivers' efforts.

In other activities of the Families and Health Care Project at the United Hospital Fund, we have already experienced the power of a fresh perspective on caregiving. Early on, we asked Peter Arno, a health economist at Montefiore Medical Center, to work with us on creating the first estimate of the economic value of informal family caregivers. The analysis, based on data from different national population-based surveys, resulted in an estimate for 1996 of $196 billion—more than the cost of formal home care and nursing home care combined and the equivalent of almost 20 percent of total health care expenditures (Arno, Levine, and Memmott 1999). In updated projections for 2000, the value had grown to $257 billion (Arno 2002). This study's findings immediately resonated with advocates, researchers, and even policymakers, who have used the summary conclusions freely to support the need for assisting family caregivers. The dollar figure itself is staggering, but even more powerful was the restatement of what family caregivers do in terms that carry weight in our society—in that case, money.

We need to develop a similarly fresh perspective on what it is that caregivers do. If we continue to use measures that we know are both imprecise and insensitive to a complex reality, we will not marshal the resources needed to assist caregivers. If we can successfully reframe the way caregiving is defined and measured, so that the dimensions of its scope and impact are better understood, we can move ahead with the hard work of designing more responsive services, educational programs, and public policies. This book is a start toward that goal.

The immediate impetus for the project that led to this book, supported in part by the Robert Wood Johnson Foundation, was the collaboration of the United Hospital Fund with the Harvard School of Public Health and the Visiting Nurse Service of New York (VNSNY) on a national and New York City random telephone survey of family caregivers, funded by the Kaiser Family Foundation and (for the New York City sample) by the Fund and VNSNY. As we collaborated in the design of the survey, we learned just how hard it is, in the limited time available in a telephone survey, to move beyond the conventional questions covered by ADLs and IADLs. We quickly understood that important elements of caregiving were ignored by these iconic measures, and that they distorted much of the reality that we sought to capture.

Despite our frustration with the ADL and IADL measures, the survey elicited information about several important but little-studied issues, especially caregivers' relationship with the formal medical care system. Guided by research conducted by the United Hospital Fund (Levine 1998), the survey attempted to learn more about the transition from hospital to home-based care. Alert to the often hurried and inadequate discharge process, the survey asked family caregivers what sources (if any) of training they had received to prepare them to perform complex medical tasks as well as to assist with ADLs. It also asked who provided the training. Understanding that rapid transitions do not define the full caregiving experience, which for many families is a long-term commitment, caregivers were also asked about their interactions with staff of the formal health care system. The survey also tried to explore caregiver perceptions of needs that were not met by the formal care system and their understanding of why these needs remained unmet.

The New York City survey findings are reported in Levine et al. (2000) and the national findings in Donelan et al. (2002). The significance of this survey for the current project is not any particular finding but its confirmation of how limited the ADL and IADL measures are for acquiring the information we wanted and how difficult it is to devise a new measurement paradigm. There were no alternative measures or measurement strategies that we could turn to, and that sparked our interest in fielding a project that would begin to reframe the issue.

Having completed the initial phase of what will certainly be a long and complex undertaking, we look next to four areas that call for further exploration and experimentation: research, professional education, public and caregiver education, and public policy.

Research

More research is needed to devise and validate more accurate definitions of caregiver activities. Without these we can howl against the dark but do no more than continue to stumble about in it.

- As Susan Reinhard (Chapter 2) demonstrates, the application of ADLs and IADLs to family caregivers, not only to care recipients, evolved without explicit consideration of their adequacy and implications. For the future, existing caregiver surveys should be refined and new surveys developed that include tested and validated definitions of caregiver activities and roles. For example, surveys should probe about a wider range of medically oriented caregiver activities, such as changing bandages, monitoring equipment, managing pain, and the like. Given the dramatic increase in polypharmacy and its attendant complexities and risks, much more information is needed about caregivers' roles and difficulties obtaining, paying for, administering, and monitoring side effects of medications.

- Steven Albert (Chapter 4) proposes a new framework for categorizing caregiving tasks. He considers timing, caregiver proximity, effort, and participation of the care recipient important determinants of the degree of difficulty of the task. In the proposed scheme, these features are arrayed against a new organizational grouping— skilled nursing care, cognitive support, in-home management, and out-of-home care management. In a fully worked-out system, family caregiver situations could be scored in a way that more fully captures the reality of what caregiving entails. Refining and validating this framework—or alternatives to it that similarly seek to capture the significant domains of caregiving and how they interact—is a high priority.

- A new framework calls for a more holistic view of the caregiving experience. In our survey, many caregivers, when asked about carrying out specific tasks, reported that they were "competent" or "comfortable"; but they gave a much more negative appraisal of their comfort level when asked about caregiving overall. Carol Levine and Andrea Hart (Chapter 1) give many vivid examples of the difference between caregiver perceptions of the complex and often emotionally charged roles they play and the limiting, mechanistic quality of the ADL and IADL measures. We need to craft measures that capture these interactive and cumulative aspects of caregiving.

- More research is needed on the management aspects of family caregiving, including dealing with government agencies, insurance companies, and vendors of equipment and supplies, and especially on the interaction between home care staff—nurses, therapists, aides— and family caregivers. Much of the existing research concerns the relationship between the caregiver and care recipient; while certainly essential, this perspective ignores the often stressful relationships between the caregiver and the outside services and people involved in the family member's care.

- Research must grapple with both the commonalities and differences experienced by caregivers. While we often search for what is shared or common, an equally important area for exploration is the variable perceptions of tasks: how different people assess the difficulty of certain tasks under different circumstances. Caregivers have different strengths and limitations; yet they are typically expected to do everything and do everything equally well. Some caregivers already know how to do certain things very well; others can become competent with appropriate training; still others will never achieve competence at particular tasks but may be well suited to others. Improved measurement of caregiver strengths and capabilities, as well as inherent limitations, will be critical to all efforts to support competent, confident family caregivers. Finding alternatives for the aspects of caregiving for which they are less well suited will be essential.

- As Lynn Friss Feinberg (Chapter 3) makes clear, current methods and practices of caregiver assessment are both inadequate and erratic. Differences in methodology, nomenclature, and specific items and approaches make it virtually impossible to compare instruments. There is no consensus about how to assess family care or what should be included in a comprehensive caregiver assessment tool. Developing such a consensus should be a high priority. Clearly, caregiver-only assessments that separate the patient's needs from the caregiver's are an important goal. Assessments should take into account not only the specific situation but also the duration of caregiving and its intensity. Assessors must be sensitive to the emotional component of caregiving as well as to its more concrete aspects.

- Very little is known about the quality of care provided by family members, except when it is very bad or amazingly good. On one hand, it seems likely that, given the complexity of caregivers' responsibilities and their typically inadequate training, quality in some cases does not meet nursing or other professional standards. If errors occur with some frequency in hospitals, nursing homes, and doctors' offices, it is safe to assume that they occur at home as well. On the other hand, competent caregivers may actually exceed professional standards since they are always on the job, have sensitive antennae for changes, and have learned precisely how to care for a particular patient. We need studies that develop ways to assist caregivers in preventing errors in medication management, symptom control, and other situations that may lead to avoidable hospitalizations or trips to the Emergency Department.

- The information garnered from all these sources should be the springboard for developing new and more sensitive programs to train, support, and counsel caregivers. Researchers and practitioners should work together to bridge the gap that often delays or prevents research findings from being translated into practice. It is also important to engage caregivers themselves in helping to evaluate programs.

Professional Education

Even the best designed, most rigorous research studies will not change practice unless health care and social service professionals are aware of the implications for their daily interactions with family caregivers. Education at all levels and for all disciplines should include familiarity with research findings, discussion about aspects of family caregiving, and opportunities to interact with family caregivers. There are many mechanisms to achieve these goals. Ideally, material on family caregiving should be included in curriculums of medical, nursing, social work, psychology, and allied health professional schools. The curricular material can be supplemented by home visits, writing assignments, and other techniques. Students usually welcome these experiences and often find them among the most rewarding of their training. It is sometimes harder to convince educators that there should be time in busy schedules for this material.

Instilling an awareness of family caregivers early in the educational process is essential, but continuing education for professionals on the job is also important. In the United Hospital Fund Family Caregiver Grant Initiative, our hospital grantees found that reaching professionals was not an easy task and called for creative techniques. Appealing to staff as family caregivers themselves, rather than as part of their job responsibilities, proved successful in several hospitals (Levine 2003).

Project DOCC (Delivery of Chronic Care), a parent-sponsored organization now working in partnership with the United Hospital Fund, is a promising model for professional training (Hoffman and Appel 2004). This project grew out of the efforts of parents of ill or disabled children to communicate to pediatricians-in-training the realities of their lives—not just the medical aspects but life at home, in school, and in the community. The program, operating now in 28 hospitals, uses family faculty to present grand rounds; home visits with the parent of the disabled child and an additional parent; and extensive, sociomedical interviews. Project DOCC's creators are now working to expand the model to caregivers of older adults.

New educational requirements set forth by the Accreditation Council for Graduate Medical Education that aim to prepare physicians to better understand and communicate with their patients and families afford a real opportunity and leverage for the implementation of this type of training program. It is also important that all the members of interdisciplinary care teams receive training in working more effectively with family caregivers.

Public and Caregiver Education

Public education is an essential part of changing the environment in which family caregiving goes on. As long as the general public (including caregivers) thinks of caregiving as "just what families do," not as a complex responsibility, it will be difficult to marshal resources and support for the kinds of specific training and assistance caregivers need. Many caregivers do not obtain even the modest assistance currently available because they do not identify themselves as caregivers (Dobrof and Ebenstein 2004). Public education can take many forms: television (which tends toward the unusual case and the emotional story), articles in newspapers and periodicals, community forums, discussions in religious settings, and volunteer activities. Broad public support is necessary for public policy changes that more fully meet caregiver needs.

Public Policy

Bruce Vladeck (Chapter 5) strikes a cautionary note: if research and practice are not fully conversant with the realities of family caregiving, public policy for the most part is even further behind. Pessimistic about the long-term prospects for revamping family caregiver policies and support, he nevertheless offers several specific proposals for the short term. They bear repeating here:

- Paid providers of formal in-home services should be required to consult regularly with informal caregivers about their own resources and needs, as well as those of the patient.
- Medicare- and Medicaid-paid home care services, for which formal patient assessments are already required, should strengthen and expand the assessment of caregiver capabilities and needs.
- Caregiver assessments should be a mandatory part of the patient assessment process for Medicaid home- and community-based waivers.
- Medicare and Joint Commission for the Accreditation of Healthcare Organizations standards for hospital discharge planning should be strengthened to require caregiver assessment, using a standard instrument, and the results incorporated into the discharge plan.

The United Hospital Fund's work on transitions from hospital to home (Levine et al. 2000), and work in progress on the transition from formal home care to total family responsibility, supports the need for the final recommendation. Here the regulatory and accreditation structures are already in place; what are needed are the resources and incentives to implement standards that address the needs of family caregivers.

In a health care environment beset with budgetary woes, personnel shortages, and increasingly high-tech yet fragmented care, it is easy to dismiss the possibility of real change. But, given the pervasiveness and centrality of family caregiving, a vigorous, sustained effort to better define and measure what caregivers do, and to understand just how important it is to the health care system, may prove to be the lever with which we can move what appears to be unmovable. With this book and these recommendations, and others that may grow out of a thoughtful consideration of these chapters, we hope that the movement, however preliminary, has begun.

References

Arno, PS. 2002, February. Economic value of informal caregiving. Paper presented at the meeting of the American Association for Geriatric Psychiatry, Orlando, FL.

Arno, PS, C Levine, and M Memmott. 1999. The economic value of informal caregiving. *Health Affairs* 18(2):182–88.

Dobrof J and H Ebenstein. 2004. Family caregiver self-identification: Implications for health care and social service professionals. *Generations*. In press.

Donelan K, CA Hill, C Hoffman, K Scoles, PH Feldman, C Levine, and D Gould. 2002. Challenged to care: Informal caregivers in a changing health system. *Health Affairs* 21(4):222–31.

Hoffman M and DJ Appel. 2004. Project DOCC: A parent-directed model for educating pediatric residents. In *The Cultures of caregiving: Conflict and common ground among families, health professionals, and policy makers*, ed. C Levine, 147–54. Baltimore: Johns Hopkins University Press.

Levine C. 1998. *Rough crossings: Family caregivers' odysseys through the health care system*. New York: United Hospital Fund.

———. 2003. *Making room for family caregivers: Seven innovative hospital programs*. New York: United Hospital Fund.

Levine C, AN Kuerbis, DA Gould, M Navaie-Waliser, PH Feldman, and K Donelan. 2000. *A survey of family caregivers in New York City: Findings and implications for the health care system*. New York: United Hospital Fund.

Family Caregivers on the Job: Moving beyond ADLs and IADLs

Carol Levine, Susan C. Reinhard, Lynn Friss Feinberg, Steven Albert, and Andrea Hart

Ask any professional in the field of aging what family caregivers do and the answer is likely to be, they help an elderly or ill person with ADLs and IADLs. In the prevailing paradigm, the caregiver's assistance compensates for the care recipient's difficulty performing one or more of the "activities of daily living," a term used to refer to such basic endeavors as bathing or using the toilet, or the "instrumental activities of daily living," referring to shopping, transportation, and the like. What the family caregiver does is assumed, at least implicitly, to be the mirror image of the care recipient's limitations.

According to Feldman and Kane (2003), ADLs are "probably the single most important research-based concept underpinning [long-term care] . . . in many respects equivalent to Freud's work in establishing a conceptual framework in psychiatry" (pp. 184–5). It is daunt-

This chapter first appeared in *Generations: Journal of the American Society on Aging* 27(4):17–23, in an issue devoted to "Family Caregiving: Current Challenges for a Time-Honored Practice," edited by Carol Levine. Work on the article, and the project from which it was drawn, was supported by a grant from the Robert Wood Johnson Foundation.

ing to challenge, however humbly, the concept that in the world of long-term care is the equivalent of the Freudian fundamentals. Nevertheless, we believe that in today's world, measures of ADLs and IADLs, which were designed to describe care recipients' limitations, do not convey the full spectrum or degree of complexity of the family caregiver's responsibilities. Yet, because ADL and IADL needs are often used or proposed as thresholds for benefits and services, standards of incorporating them have significant implications for families and for public policy. And although several researchers have described caregiving much more broadly, their contributions have not been incorporated into usual practice or policy.

The Evolution of ADLs and IADLs

Measurement of ADLs was developed in the late 1950s to describe functioning—and functional limitations—of ill or disabled older adults. Katz and colleagues (1963) developed a measure of six ADLs (bathing, dressing, using the toilet, transferring [from bed to chair, for example], continence, and feeding) to study results of treatment and prognosis in older adults hospitalized with hip fractures (and, later, other diagnoses like cerebral infarction and multiple sclerosis).

To supplement measurement of ADLs, Lawton and Brody (1969) created a measure of eight "instrumental activities of daily living" or IADLs. Many older adults might be independent in all ADLs but not able to function independently in the community because they cannot shop, cook meals, perform housework, do laundry, handle money, manage transportation, use the telephone, or take medications on their own. Lawton and Brody's IADL measure was designed to assist in developing a care plan and aid in teaching and training helping professionals.

Since the 1970s more than forty ADL and IADL measurement instruments have been developed (Feinstein, Josephy, and Wells, 1986); Robert Kane and Rosalie Kane (2000) provide reviews of the most commonly used. Despite almost universal acceptance of these instruments, measurement errors and difficulties in comparability arise with their use, even among the population for which they were originally intended (Weiner et al., 1990; Mathiowetz and Lair, 1994). While in the literature researchers specify which measures they use, in policy forums these distinctions are usually lost, and ADL and IADL measures are conflated into the simplest version.

Use of ADL and IADL measures moved from research on older adults to research on family caregiving in the 1980s and 1990s (Farran, 2001). Early studies focused on the "burden" that families experience in caring for an ill or disabled family member (see Gaugler, Kane, and Langois, 2000 for a current review of instruments to measure burden). Perhaps the most influential work linking ADLs and IADLs to family caregiving comes from the conceptualization of family caregiving as a stressful experience by Pearlin and colleagues (1990). These authors hypothesized that the care recipient's need for help with ADLs and IADLs is one of the primary objective stressors (or care demands) that lead to such effects on caregivers as depression, feelings of burden, and declines in physical health. Most caregiving research using community-based samples has drawn upon this model (Gaugler, Zarit, and Pearlin, 1999).

The broad acceptance of functional measures by gerontological researchers led researchers in the public policy arena to adopt ADL and IADL measures in national survey instruments such as the National Long-Term Care Survey of Medicare Beneficiaries and its informal caregiver supplements (Clark, 1998). From there it was an easy—and simplistic—public-policy step to link family caregivers' responsibilities to the functional deficits of their older relatives.

Family Caregivers' Perspectives

In some ways any focus on tasks misses the core of family caregiving. As Abel (1990) points out, "The chores that family and friends perform do not exist in a vacuum; rather, they are embedded in intimate personal relationships . . ." (p. 141). Jansson and colleagues (2001) contend that the "activities of daily living or instrumental care . . . divert attention from much work caregivers are engaged in and render them invisible" (p. 805). For this reason, Schumacher and her colleagues (2000) assert that caregiving should not be defined solely in terms of tasks and procedures. Nevertheless, we cannot understand the whole experience of caregiving unless we accurately describe what caregivers do, and how that varies in different situations.

The spectrum of family caregiving includes tasks that are very modest and relatively unchallenging and also tasks that are identical to nursing home care and in some instances even to hospital care. Although for some caregiving situations the ADL-IADL measures are "good enough," they do not address the scope and complexity of many caregivers' responsibilities, which include medical, coordination, and management tasks that early long-term-care researchers could not have anticipated. Caregivers do not think of what they do in terms of performing tasks related to ADLs and IADLs; they do whatever needs to be done. Then they watch and wait until the next thing needs to be done, and the next, and the next.

Bathing and Other ADLs

To take just one example of an activity included in all ADL scales, consider bathing, one of the two ADLs (using the toilet is the other) most likely to be accompanied by all other ADLs and by IADLs as well (Levine et al., 2000). For an ill or disabled person, bathing is an important health measure to prevent infection, a formerly pleasurable activity, and also has social implications (because it controls body odor) (Sloane et al., 1995). Yet bathing is clearly one of the most difficult tasks, particularly if the care recipient has dementia or mobility problems (Rader and Barrick, 2000).

The caregiver may encounter disruptive behavior, particularly when the care recipient feels confused, threatened, or insulted, or if he or she is physically uncomfortable. The care recipient may perceive certain acts, like being moved into the bathroom, undressed, and washed, as physical or sexual abuse and may respond with combative behavior. If the care recipient suffers from arthritis or other mobility problems, he or she may resist going into the bathroom because movement is painful.

Even when the care recipient is more passive, bathing can present difficult challenges. Because the body deteriorates and loses its resiliency and elasticity with age, an older person's bones are more prone to fractures and breaks. One caregiver reported the following: "My father had no muscles. Coarse skin covered bones that were held together by tendons that seemed frayed and rigid. I was afraid that I would pull off a limb if I lifted him wrong" (Pisetsky, 1998, p. 869). There are, of course, many ways to avoid or reduce these anxieties, but most caregivers are not given any training to perform tasks related to ADLs (Levine et al., 2000).

Moreover, most private homes are not like hospitals or nursing homes, which have special facilities for showers. Whatever a caregiver has observed or been taught in such a facility is not easy to replicate at home. The level of difficulty in bathing a home-bound person is often equal to that of bathing a nursing home resident, acknowledged as a complex task for which training is necessary (Rader and Barrick, 2000).

Shopping and Other IADLs

Compared to the intense, intimate, and often demanding physical nature of tasks related to ADLs, helping a person perform IADLs may seem easy. In some situations no special training or adaptations are required, and the emotional component of caregiving is minimized. However, even IADL tasks that do not present big challenges individually can collectively take a great deal of the caregiver's time (Bakas, Lewis, and Parsons, 2001) and require lifestyle adjustments. One male caregiver wrote, "The first week was a crisis period for me, since I felt that I had to juggle a host of obligations and responsibilities. It had come on more suddenly than I had expected . . . regular meals had to be provided, visits to the doctor, spending time and [keeping him] occup[ied] . . ." (Schindler, 1996, pp. 6–7).

Of all the IADLs, shopping seems the least problematic. However, many of the items the care recipient needs—special, often expensive, foods or incontinence supplies, not to mention assistive devices—are not ones that consumers typically buy or know where to find. If the family's overall budget is limited, then the family caregiver has to set priorities about the purchase of particular items.

Getting from place to place and making telephone calls are also IADLs. A survey of caregivers of patients with lung cancer found that adult children rated transportation as the most time-consuming task, while spouses rated it as the second (providing emotional support was first) (Bakas, Lewis, and Parsons, 2001). When an elderly or cognitively impaired person does not have the functional capacity to operate a telephone (look up numbers, dial, and answer the phone), it is the family caregiver who initiates calls or answers the phone. If telephone calls were limited to chats with friends and family or other routine calls, life would be relatively simple. Most caregivers view making telephone calls as extended and repeated interventions on behalf of the family member. Many of these calls are to healthcare professionals, to schedule appointments, check on test results, report symptoms, or reorder prescriptions. Many are to navigate the labyrinths of reimbursement for healthcare costs and equipment from public or private sources.

As hospital stays have become shorter and more homecare technology has become available, caregiving at home has come to take on many of the aspects of a mini intensive-care unit. Caregivers may find themselves providing care unassisted in a situation that requires more clinical skills than are ordinarily expected of lay people (Schumacher et al., 2000). Such is particularly the case with medication management. When the IADL measures were constructed, managing medications was generally fairly simple. Now, however, the pharmaceutical armamentarium is enormous and complex. Medications are administered not only orally, but also by IV, suppository, and aerosol. Travis, Bethea, and Win (2000) categorized medication administration "hassles" into three main categories: scheduling logistics, administration procedures, and safety issues (medication errors).

What the ADL/IADL Measures Miss about Caregiving

Family caregiving encompasses several complex activities embedded in but not formally recognized by ADL-IADL measures. The primary activity of this kind is provision of emotional support (Bakas, Lewis, and Parsons, 2001), which is the expression of the caregiver's love and concern that are the usual motivations for assuming the caregiving role. Depending on the situation, caregivers also engage in gathering information on homecare services; monitoring and supervising the care recipient's behavior; managing medical equipment and providing skilled nursing care, including managing pain symptoms; managing hired care professionals or paraprofessionals; making decisions about treatment and place of care; and acting throughout as the care recipient's agent and advocate. One caregiver reported, "You're a banker, an emotional confidant, a friend, a medical advocate. . . . You're dealing with medicines, the medical bureaucracy, trying to find housing. You have to have an expertise in more than you can possibly know about—that's why people need help" (McLeod, 1995, p. 1).

Behavior Supervision

Probably the most extensively described caregiver task not included in the basic ADL-IADL measures is monitoring and supervising the behavior of patients with dementia (Jansson, Nordberg, and Grafstrom, 2001). Performing all the ADL-IADL tasks becomes more complicated when the care recipient is frightened or hostile. Even without the physiological changes associated with dementia, many people do not adapt easily to illness. They may express their anger and frustration at their dependence by lashing out at the caregiver or others in the home.

High-Tech Homecare

High-tech homecare is a relatively recent phenomenon. Before the 1980s most kinds of medical care involving medical equipment were limited to in-patient settings and delivered and monitored by professional staff. Today high-tech homecare is a big business, and almost anything that can be done in an intensive care unit can be done at home, including artificial nutrition and hydration, mechanical ventilation, maintaining heart function, and infusion therapies. Although high-tech equipment has many benefits, it also presents many challenges to the family caregiver. Caregivers of people using home ventilation reported feeling "tied" by home medical equipment (Moss et al., 1993; Van Kesteren, Velthuis, and van Leyden, 2001) because regular suctioning is required to prevent the patient from choking, and the caregiver has to be on call to respond to alarms.

Pain Management

Pain control is still one of the least well managed aspects of professional medical care. Yet untrained family caregivers are routinely given the responsibility of managing pain at home. Ferrell (2001) asserts that "family caregivers who have very little information about pharmacology, dosing of medications, and assessing or treating pain are asked to become the 24-hour-a-day care providers" (p. 596). She adds the following:

> The professional's task of spending a few minutes with a patient in pain and then to be able to go home at the end of the day is very different from living 24 hours a day, seven days a week for years on end with someone in pain. . . . Dealing with regulatory barriers from a family perspective means that you must travel farther to get prescriptions refilled, you must go to different pharmacies, and you

must take your loved one to multiple doctors to get the necessary medications. (p. 596)

Managing Paid Homecare Workers

Although some homecare services provide limited assistance, their presence does not decrease the amount of informal care provided (Caro and Stern, 1995). On the contrary, the presence of paid help presents another managerial responsibility, as "adult children find themselves operating like personnel managers for their ailing parents, having to recruit workers, check references, set wages and supervise" (McLeod, 1995, p. 1).

Advocacy in Negotiating the Healthcare System

Advocacy is necessary because the medical-care system has become increasingly fragmented and complicated; a physician is not always accessible or available and is not always aware of what is happening day-to-day with a particular patient. Trying to advocate in behalf of the care recipient can be frustrating to the caregiver, particularly when physicians and other healthcare professionals fail to keep the caregiver informed about the care recipient's health. Care partners report frequent problems with their level of participation and their communication with providers (vom Eigen et al., 1999).

Even health professionals who become caregivers may find themselves helpless: A social worker reported, "I quickly came to understand how powerless even I . . . was in negotiating decisions concerning [my mother's] medical care" (Anonymous, 2000, p. 1).

Current Approaches to Caregiver Assessment

One of the advantages of the ADL-IADL measures is that they provide a quick, albeit truncated, snapshot of an individual's level of impairment and a broad, albeit sketchy, outline of the needed assistance. Starting with an ADL-IADL baseline, many caregiver assessments have been developed, although most have been developed for research rather than everyday practice and care management. [See Lynn Friss Feinberg's article in this issue.] A Canadian research team that surveyed sixty-three caregiver assessment tools found that none of the validated tools addressed a range of caregiver issues or specified caregivers' service needs (Guberman et al., 2001a and 2001b; Fancey and Keefe, 1999).

Thirty-four of the sixty-three tools were general assessments, usually designed to determine eligibility for homecare or support services. They focused on the willingness, ability, and capacity of the caregiver to continue providing care—from the perspective of the assessor, not the caregiver. Although some assessments asked the care recipient about the needs of the caregiver, generally these tools did not ask caregivers to assess their own needs and emotional health or allow the caregivers to provide their perspective of the situation. The twenty-nine caregiver-specific assessment tools asked a variety of questions about tasks and burdens.

The National Family Caregiver Support Program, the first federal program designed specifically to support caregiver services, does not mandate caregiver assessment. Prior to its enactment, some states established state-funded caregiver support programs. While the majority of state programs use some form of assessment to determine eligibility or develop a care plan, most publicly funded programs do not uniformly or systematically assess the needs and situation of the family caregiver (Feinberg and Pilisuk, 1999; Feinberg, 2002).

Expanding the Domains of Family Caregiving

What is needed is a broader conceptual framework for the domains of family caregiving that reframes and supplements traditional tasks by taking into account family caregiver perspectives as well as the aspects of care not adequately covered in ADLs and IADLs. Table 1 suggests such a scheme. (A fuller explanation of this model appears in Albert, 2004.)

Table 1
Expanded Caregiving Domains

Direct Care Provision	Care Management
• ADL Care	• In-Home Care Management
• Skilled Nursing Care	• Out-of-Home Care Management
• Cognitive Support	

Within a framework of two basic types of care, direct care provision includes ADL care, skilled nursing care (wound care, medication management, equipment operation), and cognitive support (behavior supervision, monitoring, and cuing). Care management is divided into in-home and out-of-home activities. In-home care management includes activities such as home modification; hiring and supervision of homecare aides; and purchase, maintenance, and upkeep of assistive devices. Out-of-homecare management includes activities such as arranging for medical care, processing insurance claims, transportation, and financial management.

Within these domains four key contextual features determine how families deliver care (Table 2). One feature is timing: whether care is required rarely, frequently but in predictable ways, or frequently in unpredictable ways (Montgomery, Gonyea, and Hooyman, 1985).

A second dimension is caregiver proximity. Is it enough that a caregiver is in the house while someone eats a meal or bathes, or does the caregiver need to be in the same room standing by, or does the caregiver have to provide hands-on help?

Table 2
Contextual Features of a Caregiving Domain

Timing	Caregiver Proximity	Caregiver Effort	Care Receiver Response
• Occasional	• Stand-by	• Coaxing	• Cooperative
• Frequent	• Hands-on	• Guiding	• Passive
Predictable		• Controlling	• Obstructive
Unpredictable			

A third difference is the kind of effort caregivers need to exert to see that the need is met. Someone with a need for help in bathing may only require supervision, or coaxing and support, or complete guidance and direction. Finally, the behaviors of care recipients matter. They may participate fully, actively resist, or passively accept care (Feinstein, Josephy, and Wells, 1986).

In each of the domains and subdomains of care (such as the components of ADL care), appropriate distinctions can be made along the axes of timing, proximity, caregiver effort, and care-recipient response. A next step would be to devise a scoring system that would more accurately represent the caregiver's responsibilities. Such a system would enable practitioners and researchers to understand more clearly why families taking care of relatives with the same number of ADLs and IADLs differ in their experiences of adapting to the challenges and need different types of support.

In conclusion, family caregivers of the twenty-first century face different challenges from their counterparts of the mid-twentieth century. Research, practice, and policy must adapt to help them meet these challenges. The development, validation, and implementation of refinements and supplements to ADL/IADL measures would be an important step in that direction.

References

Abel, E.K. 1990. "Informal Care for the Disabled Elderly: A Critique of Recent Literature." *Research on Aging* 12(2): 139–57.

Albert, S.M. 2004. "Beyond ADL/IADL: Recognizing the Full Scope of Family Caregiving." In Levine, C., ed. *Family Caregivers on the Job: Moving Beyond ADLs and IADLS.* New York: United Hospital Fund.

Anonymous. 2000. "Outrageous: Our Society is Just Not Ready." *Alzheimer's Association Newsletter, New York Chapter.* Summer: 1, 5, 12. Available at www. alzheimernyc.org/Newsletter/newsletter.htm. (Accessed January 19, 2004.)

Bakas, T., Lewis, R.R., and Parsons, J.E. 2001. "Caregiving Tasks Among Family Caregivers of Patients with Lung Cancer." *Oncology Nursing Forum* 28(5): 847–54.

Caro, F.G., and Stern, A.L. 1995. "Balancing Formal and Informal Care: Meeting Need in a Resource-Constrained Program." *Home Health Care Services Quarterly* 15(4): 67–81.

Clark, R. 1998. "An Introduction to the National Long-Term Care Surveys." From http://aspe.os.dhhs.gov/daltcp/reports/nltcssu2.htm. (Accessed Feb. 25, 2003).

Fancey, P., and Keefe, J.M. 1999. *Development of Screening and Assessment Tools for Family Caregivers. Phase I Report on Review of Nonvalidated Tools.* Nova Scotia, Canada: Mount St. Vincent University.

Farran, C. 2001. "Family Caregiver Intervention Research: Where Have We Been? Where Are We Going?" *Journal of Gerontological Nursing* 27(7): 38–45.

Feinberg, L.F. 2002. *The State of the Art: Caregiver Assessment in Practice Settings.* San Francisco: Family Caregiver Alliance.

Feinberg, L.F., and Pilisuk, T.L. 1999. *Survey of Fifteen States Caregiver Support Programs: Final Report.* San Francisco: Family Caregiver Alliance.

Feinstein, A.R., Josephy, B.R., and Wells, C.K. 1986. "Scientific and Clinical Problems in Indexes of Functional Disability." *Annals of Internal Medicine* 105: 413–20.

Feldman, P.H. and Kane, R.L. 2003. "Strengthening Research to Improve the Practice and Management of Long-term Care." *The Milbank Quarterly* 81(2): 179–220.

Ferrell, B. 2001. "Pain Observed: The Experience of Pain from the Family Caregiver's Perspective." *Clinics in Geriatric Medicine* 17(3): 595–609.

Gaugler, J.E., Kane, R.A., and Langlois, J. 2000. "Assessment of Family Caregivers of Older Adults." In R.L. Kane and R.A. Kane, eds., *Assessing Older Persons: Measures, Meaning, and Practical Applications* (pp. 320–359). New York: Oxford University Press.

Gaugler, J.E., Zarit, S.H., and Pearlin, L.I. 1999. "Caregiving and Institutionalization: Perceptions of Family Conflict and Sociometric Support." *International Journal of Aging and Human Development* 49(1): 1–25.

Guberman, N., et al. 2001a. *Assessment Tools Serving the Needs of Caregivers: A Document to Better Understand the Importance of Assessing Caregivers' Needs.* Montreal, Canada: School of Social Work, University of Quebec at Montreal.

Guberman, N., et al. 2001b. *Development of Screening and Assessment Tools for Family Caregivers: Final Report.* Montreal, Canada: School of Social Work, University of Quebec at Montreal.

Jansson, W., Nordberg, G., and Grafstrom, M. 2001. "Patterns of Elderly Spousal Caregiving in Dementia Care: An Observational Study." *Journal of Advanced Nursing* 34(6): 804–12.

Kane, R.L., and Kane, R.A., eds., 2000. *Assessing Older Persons: Measuring, and Practical Applications.* New York: Oxford University Press.

Katz, S. et al. 1963. "Studies of Illness in the Aged: The Index of ADL: A Standardized Measure of Biological and Psychosocial Function." *Journal of the American Medical Association* 185(12): 94–9.

Lawton, M.P., and Brody, E.M. 1969. "Assessment of Older People: Self-maintaining and Instrumental Activities of Daily Living." *The Gerontologist* 9(3): 179–86.

Levine, C., et al. 2000. *A Survey of Family Caregivers in New York City: Findings and Implications for the Health Care System.* New York: United Hospital Fund.

McLeod, B.W. 1995. "No Place Like Home." *San Francisco Examiner*, April 3, 1995, p. 1.

Mathiowetz, N.A., and Lair, T.J. 1994. "Getting Better? Change or Error in the Measurement of Functional Limitations." *Journal of Economic and Social Measurement* 20: 237–62.

Montgomery, R.J.V., Gonyea, J.G., and Hooyman, N.R. 1985. "Caregiving and the Experience of Subjective and Objective Burden." *Family Relations* 34: 19–26.

Moss, A.H., et al. 1993. "Home Ventilation for Amyotrophic Lateral Sclerosis Patients: Outcomes, Costs, and Patient, Family, and Physician Attitudes." *Neurology* 43: 438–43.

Pearlin, L.I., Mullan, J.T., Semple, S.J., and Skaff, M.M. 1990. "Caregiving and the Stress Process: An Overview of Concepts and Their Measures." *The Gerontologist* 30: 583–94.

Pisetsky, D.S. 1998. "Doing Everything." *Annals of Internal Medicine* 128(10): 869–70.

Rader, J., and Barrick, A.L. 2000. "Ways That Work: Bathing Without a Battle." *Alzheimer's Care Quarterly* 1(4):35–49.

Rodgers, W., and Miller, B. 1997. "A Comparative Analysis of ADL Questions in Surveys of Older People." *The Journal of Gerontology* 52B:21–36.

Schindler, R. 1996. "Normative Crises of the Very Old and Their Adult Children: A Personal Account." *Journal of Gerontological Social Work* 25(3/4): 3–15.

Schumacher, K.L. et al. 2000. "Family Caregiving Skill: Development of the Concept." *Research in Nursing & Health* 23:191–203.

Sloane, P.D., et al. 1995. "Bathing Persons with Dementia." *The Gerontologist* 35(5): 672–8.

Travis, S.S., Bethea, L.S., and Winn, P. 2000. "Medication Administration Hassles Reported by Family Caregivers of Dependent Elderly Persons." *Journal of Gerontology* 55A(7):M412–17.

van Kesteren, R.G., Velthuis, B., and van Leyden, L.W. 2001. "Psychosocial Problems Arising from Home Ventilation." *American Journal of Physical Medicine & Rehabilitation* 80(6): 439–46.

vom Eigen, K.A., et al. 1999. "Care Partner Experiences with Hospital Care." *Medical Care* 37(1): 33–8.

Weiner, J.M., et al.1990. "Measuring the Activities of Daily Living: Comparisons across National Surveys." *Journal of Gerontology* 45(6): S229–37.

About the Authors

Steven M. Albert, PhD, MS, is associate professor of clinical public health in the Department of Sociomedical Sciences at Columbia University's Mailman School of Public Health and the Gertrude H. Sergievsky Center and Department of Neurology at Columbia University College of Physicians and Surgeons. He is trained as an anthropologist and epidemiologist. Dr. Albert's research centers on the functional significance of cognitive deficit and its broader impact on health outcomes and subjective reports of quality of life. He has published over 50 papers in this area, as well as two books. He has carried this research forward in the areas of HIV-related dementia, Alzheimer's disease, and most recently in non-demented older adults. He has also begun a series of studies designed to understand patient and family decision-making in chronic neurologic disease.

Lynn Friss Feinberg is deputy director of the National Center on Caregiving at the San Francisco-based Family Caregiver Alliance. The Center works to advance the development of high-quality, cost-effective policies and programs for caregivers in every state in the country. Currently, she is directing a 50-state survey, funded by the U.S. Administration on Aging, to profile "The State of the States in Family Caregiver Support." In recent years, her research has also focused on choice and decision-making for persons with cognitive impairment and their family caregivers. She now serves as co-investigator for a longitudinal study, funded by the National Institute of Mental Health, to develop interventions for caregiver mental health. Prior to 2001, Ms. Feinberg was FCA's Director of Research and Information Programs. Previous positions include serving as area agency on aging planner and evaluator, and conducting aging policy research at the University of California, San Francisco.

David A. Gould is senior vice president for program at the United Hospital Fund, where he is responsible for the Fund's grants programs; for the senior management of its program development, policy analysis, and health services research staff; and for the direction of the Fund's conference activities. He has guided the development of the Fund's major program initiatives, including palliative care, family caregiving, primary care development, and aging-in-place. In addition to having participated in leadership commissions responsible for developing policy recommendations on a range of health care issues, he currently chairs the National Advisory Committee of the Center to Advance Palliative Care at the Mount Sinai School of Medicine.

Andrea Hart is a program associate in the United Hospital Fund's Division of Education and Program Initiatives, where she manages and coordinates research and programmatic activities for the Families and Health Care Project.

Carol Levine directs the United Hospital Fund's Families and Health Care Project. She was director of the Citizens Commission on AIDS in New York City from 1987 to 1991 and director of the Orphan Project from 1991 to 1996. As a senior staff associate of The Hastings Center, she edited the *Hastings Center Report*. In 1993 she was awarded a MacArthur Foundation Fellowship for her work in AIDS policy and ethics. She has written and edited several books and articles, including a "Sounding Board" essay in the *New England Journal of Medicine* entitled "The Loneliness of the Long-Term Care Giver," *Always On Call: When Illness Turns Families into Caregivers* (2004), *Making Room for Family Caregivers: Seven Innovative Hospital Programs* (2003), and *The Cultures of Caregiving: Conflict and Common Ground among Families, Health Professionals and Policy Makers* (2004).

Susan C. Reinhard, PhD, MSN, is the co-director of the Rutgers Center for State Health Policy, a policy research center founded to stimulate sound and creative state health policy in New Jersey and around the nation. She serves as deputy commissioner of the New Jersey Department of Health and Senior Services. She also directs two national initiatives to provide policy analysis and technical support to states. She is the director of the Community Living Exchange Collaborative at Rutgers, assisting states funded by the Centers for Medicare and Medicaid Services to design long-term care systems that help people with disabilities live in their homes and communities. She is also the national program director of the Robert Wood Johnson Foundation's "State Solutions" program to help states enroll more low-income older adults and people with disabilities in the Medicare Savings Programs.

Bruce C. Vladeck is professor of health policy and geriatrics at the Mount Sinai School of Medicine in New York. From 1993 through 1997, Dr. Vladeck was Administrator of the Health Care Financing Administration (HCFA) of the U.S. Department of Health and Human Services. Before joining the federal government, Dr. Vladeck served ten years as president of the United Hospital Fund of New York. He has also held positions on the faculty of Columbia University, at the Robert Wood Johnson Foundation, and, from 1979 through 1982, as assistant commissioner of the New Jersey State Department of Health. Dr. Vladeck has published widely, perhaps most notably in his book, *Unloving Care: The Nursing Home Tragedy* (1980).

Index